THE FALL AND THE RISE

THE FALL AND THE RISE

A Teacher's Own Journey
Following A Traumatic Brain Injury

FIROZA QURESHI

Copyright © 2020 Firoza Qureshi

ISBN: 978-1-7770969-0-8

*Dedicated to my loving parents who gave me life
and they always be in my heart and mind*

*And for my husband Vikar, my pillar in gloomy season who
supported me to stand strongly at gloomy weather.*

*And for my son Sharon, my backbone in all seasons
who gave me strongest motivation.*

And all family and friends for biggest comfort.

My Loving Parents

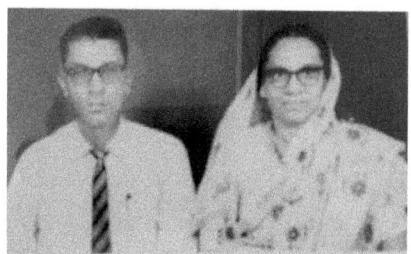

CONTENTS

Introduction ix
Preface xi
Author's Note xiii
Chapter 1 - Treatment at Victoria Hospital 1
Chapter 2 - The Rehabilitation at Parkwood 15
Chapter 3 - The Rising Process at Home Sweet Home 49
Acknowledgments 104

INTRODUCTION

I WAS A SCIENCE teacher and then an administrator and worked as a vice principal in Mohsin Bhai Zaveri Girls School and Junior College, Ballarpur, in India. I came to Canada in 2007. Beside completing other educational courses, I did Master of Education/M. Ed. from Western University, London, Ontario. As a professional, I initially worked as an Early Childhood Education/ECE teacher. Later, I joined Thames Valley District School Board, London, Ontario, Canada as an occasional secondary school teacher.

One day, as I was going to resume my work after the break, I fell on the stairs in the school I was working. This accident led me to a traumatic brain injury which affected my whole life. In this book, I have mentioned my experience from April 09, 2018, the day of getting injured, to November 2019, when I completed this book.

I am not a professional writer. However, I have tried to keep my language simple and expressive. In my writing I have tried not to get carried away with a flood of emotions and personal opinions.

During my hospital stay and later in my hospital visits, I have seen several patients struggling to recover. After talking to them, I realized that their problems are multi-layered – personal, physical, medical, psychological, social, and so on so forth. Unfortunately, most of them felt that they will never recover fully.

I also observed that the medical teams – doctors, nurses, therapists, health care providers, social workers, and all others – try to help the patients a lot by performing their duties with complete dedication. However, sometimes some patients ignore the help, by sinking into the worries of their own health issues.

This narration is my humble attempt to inspire the patients to remain positive towards the approach and guidance given by the medical teams. This book will become meaningful, if it inspires even one patient to be optimistic. However, I believe that such optimism will be counted as a success of the medical team and their own dedication. I do not want any credit for this book.

PREFACE

I HAVE PRESENTED HERE the account of my traumatic brain injury, followed by the process of the recovery. The narration is presented in the chronological order, in the form of a diary. However, it reveals my inner development, my thought process, and my psychological picture along with presenting my rehabilitation process.

In our lives, we all play multiple roles - personal, social, and professional. In the personal and the social fields, I have been a daughter, a sister, a mother, a wife, a friend, and a woman too. As a professional, I have been a teacher, a supervisor, and a vice principal. My different roles have brought all the relevant pieces of memories in my narration, to assist the readers in understanding the description.

The readers will find 'I', 'me', 'myself' a lot in the narration. However, my narration is not meant to keep myself in the focus by giving the importance to the 'self'. I am only a medium, and so are the recollected memories and incidents. The centre of this narration is the psychological development of a patient while going through a process of recovery.

I have mentioned almost all personalities that came in my contact during my struggling days. However, a limited narration cannot contain all characters. Thus, I apologize for missing some names and their identities here. I acknowledge that they have played a significant role in my recovery process.

As a brain injury patient, I want to share my experience with other patients. At different stages of treatment, a patient encounters several uncertainties, which are natural. However, such doubts slow down their process of recovery, and elevate their physical and mental pain. I request them to go through my narration and see if I have succeeded in sharing their feelings, emotions, and agonies that surface during their struggling period.

As a patient, my optimistic approach would lead me nowhere, if I did not have the support and the guidance of the doctors, nurses, therapists, health care providers, social workers and all other supporting staff, including the ambulance operators and taxi drivers. I am grateful for their tolerance and compassion that bear my persisting anxieties, necessities, and impatience which were the natural outcome of my then sufferings. However, I still apologize for their inconvenience, and accept that returning their favour is impossible for me. Nevertheless, if a single patient gets help from my narration, then I will think that I have made a small contribution to the noble cause of the medical teams.

AUTHOR'S NOTE

EVERY TRAUMATIC BRAIN injury is unique thus the treatment may vary. However, all recovery processes require internal motivation, dedication, the ability of relearning and problem solving on the part of the patients themselves. Above all, the patients also need potent medical support.

I am fortunate for having the top-level medical care from Victoria Hospital, London, Ontario. The hospital's timely treatment has saved my life and provided me with the much-needed medical support in overcoming the damage caused by the accident.

I am also grateful to the rehabilitation team and the medical experts from Parkwood Institute, London, Ontario, Canada. They have provided me with the medical guidance and support in achieving a positive and creative life after suffering from a traumatic brain injury.

My experience as a patient has conveyed to me that stepping into a trouble requires only one wrong step but getting out of it needs several well-planned steps. The recovery process is like collecting several blocks and building a bridge, brick by brick. This book is about the process of rehabilitation after 'the Fall', getting a traumatic brain injury and 'the Rise', building of a new life – The Fall and The Rise.

CHAPTER 1

TREATMENT AT VICTORIA HOSPITAL

"A hospital serves you, treats you, and saves your life. Paradoxically, it makes you feel to come inside when you are out of it, and to go out when you are in"

Monday, April 9, 2018:

Victoria Hospital, London, Ontario, Canada

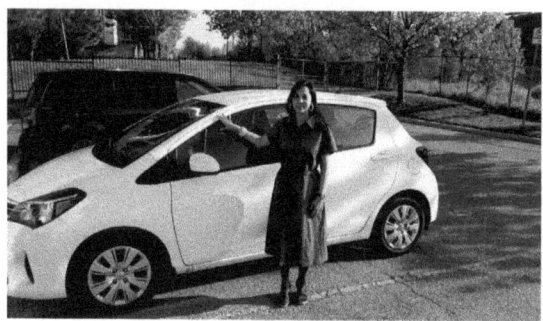

My Car

IT WAS A sunny day that could provide anyone with the clarity of vision and mind. Having no confusion or stress, I happily set out, in my Yaris, for my occasional secondary school teaching job, which was at

Montcalm Secondary School in London, Ontario, Canada. I had finished teaching my first period and had taken my break. I was talking to other teachers and collecting their experiences, feedback and suggestions. Having some enthusiastic thoughts in my mind for the next class at noon, I started descending the second-floor main stairs, and the next moment, all of the sudden, there was complete silence and deep darkness around me for the next twelve hours. All I had during those twelve hours was the collection of a few glimpses of foggy pictures and perplexing brief pieces of conversation. Later, I was given details of the series of incidents by my husband, Vikar, my son, Sharon, and doctors.

I had slipped down the stairs, got the back side of my head hit on one of the stairs, and lost my senses. The school called an ambulance that carried me to the Emergency at the Victoria Hospital. The school also informed my husband and son as to what had happened. They arrived at the hospital before 1 pm. My son tried to talk to me, like the doctors on duty, who were also asking basic questions. However, I could not respond as I was hearing only some vague voices. I had an uncomfortable neck supporter tied tightly, as the doctors suspected that I might have a neck injury too. The doctors told my husband that I might respond once I came out of the shock.

My son had to leave as he had an exam scheduled at Waterloo. My husband convinced him that I would recover, telling him how the doctors thought I might be almost fine after overcoming the shock and injury. A little bit relieved, my son left, but my husband stayed there, standing beside my bed. In the next half hour, the situation dramatically changed, when I was unable to respond much, apart from telling my name, address, date, and profession. I was also unsuccessfully trying to remove the tightly tied uncomfortable neck supporter.

The team of doctors decided to go for a head/brain scan, which was done by 4 pm, but unfortunately, the radiologist was not available. The doctors told my husband that they had only one radiologist available, and he would be in the hospital only after 6 pm. Thus, any further decision would be made only after that. They also made it clear that I was out of the danger, but they could not decline the possibility of memory and brain malfunctioning. They needed more medical tests to find a firm conclusion, however, they did me a great favour by removing the neck supporter. I was apparently fine from the front facial side, but my back of head was injured. It had a deep wound, though the bleeding had stopped.

At approximately 9 pm, the radiologist, along with other doctors, decided that it was safe to move me from the ICU/emergency area to the brain injury section, which was in another wing on the 6th floor of the same hospital. The radiologist also mentioned that a support team, comprised of a hearing analyst, physiotherapist, speech therapist and neurosurgeon would be needed for making any further decisions. That was the beginning of a long chain of diagnoses, examination, analyses, discussion, feedback, and recommendation, that started the next day.

I opened my eyes around 11 am then next day, when a nurse was adjusting my blanket. The nurse gave me some instructions, but most of them went over my head. I was not able to comprehend her voice. It appeared like her voice was coming from a dark long tunnel. I just nodded my head in order to assure her that I understood whatever she had said. I closed my eyes without any effort, and once again fell asleep.

The medical team, however, had different ideas and plans: they wanted to diagnose my mental state and the impact of injury on my cognitive capabilities, thus, it was essential that I should remain awake, and keep responding to their questions. This was very difficult for me, as I was hardly in the state to comprehend any instructions given to me or to participate in a simple and short conversation. These processes were highly energy consuming for me. Simply keeping eyes open was quite a demanding activity at that time.

The bed was comfortable, but I could not leave it or even move on it without the support of a nurse. I needed to push a bell button even for changing my posture. The washroom was attached, but again I had to call a nurse to use it. There was a closet in which my clothing was kept, however, I was in a hospital apron, and was not allowed to wear any other clothing.

The hospital staff left some food items for me, assuming I would be hungry at some point. In fact, they kept a menu card for me, and I had to select the items that I liked to eat. Since I was not comprehending anything, they brought the food by guessing my taste. My husband, too, brought some food from the cafeteria located in the lower section, but during those hours I had lost my appetite.

In the remaining day, several doctors and therapists visited and tried to ask me diagnostic questions. The questions were simple and in two categories. The basic and personal questions were about my name, profession, address, date, family members, etc. They also asked some impersonal and analytical questions, like where I was teaching the last time, what kind of vehicle I had, where the hospital is located, etc. Mostly, my answers were short and incorrect because I couldn't hear their questions properly.

The rest of the day, I went through further medical check-ups, like doing scans of my head injury, finding its impact on the body, checking blood pressure, and testing the response of my body to the given medical treatment. While going through all these medical exercises, I was feeling extremely weak, but got relieved and relaxed when I finally returned to bed. The nurse gave me some instructions, which I pretended to understand. My husband was resting on the nearby chair, but I had no energy to converse with him. He said something about the food, which I ignored and closed my eyes to fall asleep, not knowing that the next day would be even busier in terms of the diagnostic process.

The following day when I opened my eyes, I saw my husband sitting on the chair placed near the window. We were on the sixth floor, so apparently, he could get a panoramic view of the city. Such a panoramic view was something that I would have previously enjoyed a lot, however at that moment, I was unable to function mentally or physically. Enjoying the panoramic view was a far-fetched aspiration, in fact, I preferred to keep that window covered with the curtains, as I would feel uncomfortable with the heavy wind that kept banging on it.

I had my breakfast kept beside me on a trolley. The nurse told me that the attendant would come back in an hour to collect the trolley. She also told me to select the food items for the lunch from the menu.

I chose some items with her help. My mouth was not as sour as it was during the last night, but still I found the breakfast tasteless. Still, I ate some food items and drank milk. Later, on my request, my husband brought some home cooked food, which was spicier. Not only the hospital allowed it, but the nurses kept the food into the hospital fridge.

After an hour, two therapists entered the room. Their approach was assuring and friendly. They were about to diagnose my cognitive skills. I had hearing problems, which was solved by my husband. He repeated their questions loudly in different word choices. I correctly replied most of their basic questions, such as what the date it was and where the hospital was.

However, the real problem commenced when they started asking some analytical questions. I replied most of them incorrectly. For example, I was unable to reply properly the questions based on the pictures and diagrams. The real reason for my wrong answers was my partial hearing loss. I could not hear properly what they were saying. Nevertheless, I thought that I would get discharged if I replied quickly. I was under the impression that they were testing my cognitive skills and my quick replies would prove that I was physically fit to go back home. Thus, I was trying my best to pretend that I could hear properly.

Nonetheless, the medical team had different ideas and plans. They wanted to diagnose my mental state and the impact of injury on my cognitive capabilities. Thus, it was essential that I should remain awake, and keep responding to their questions. However, I was hardly in the state to comprehend any instructions given to me or to participate in a simple and short conversation. These processes were highly energy consuming for me. Simply, keeping eyes open was quite demanding activity at that time.

The entire day, the therapists kept recording my wrong answers. Finally, they expressed their concerns about my cognitive skills to my husband. To assure them, he explained that the wrong answers might be the result of my physical weakness that had a negative impact on my understanding of the questions. He was able to convince them that the next day would be better as I would be more comfortable in the hospital environment and would be recovered from the initial shock.

The next day, I had an appointment scheduled with the radiologist. He noticed my brain related issues in his first visit itself. As per the schedule, the therapists appeared on the scene before the noon with some more diagnostic activities, especially with the picture tests. My hearing capabilities were still limited though not deteriorating. Thus, my most answers were wrong. Today, my husband was not there to simplify the questions and to convey them loudly to me. Therefore, my hearing problem got seriously elevated, when I made mistakes in identifying familiar and common pictures. For instance, I could not differentiate between hippopotamus and rhinoceros. The therapists were polite with me, but I could see the signs of disagreement, disappointment, and worries over their faces.

They waited for my husband who soon came there with some food for me. They told him that they seriously felt that I had lost most of my cognitive skills and probably some part of my memory too. He was suggested to have a conversation with the radiologist, who had some information to share. The radiologist checked me in the morning and expressed his satisfaction with the process of recovery. Thus, I was certain that there was no serious issue, and I would get discharged after completing some formalities. Consequently, I kept asking my husband that when we would be able to go back home. He would keep telling me that we would be in our home in just couple of days.

After lunch, the radiologist explained to my husband that the extreme bleeding from the head wound might have affected my brain functioning capabilities. He also felt that those cognitive mistakes I was making might be the indication of serious brain damage. To make any decisive conclusion, he asked my husband about my routine activities, my working habits and other skills, including driving. My husband gave him all details. He also added that I always took some extra time to get accustomed with the new environment and situation. After listening to my husband, the doctor asked for my son's contact number, which my husband provided him. However, my husband also mentioned that my son was preparing for his exams. The doctor assured him that it would be a brief conversation and nothing negative would be conveyed to my son. To remove any possible misunderstanding, my husband informed my son that the doctor was about to contact him to seek some supplementary information. Soon, the doctor contacted my son with the same questions and my son confirmed what my husband told to the doctor.

Finally, the doctor did some medical check ups, and told me that I was recovering well, but needed to be put for some time under the medical supervision. He gave me instructions that I needed to be careful while moving my body, especially head, as there must not be any sudden movements. He also added that I was free to eat whatever I wanted or to sleep whenever I wanted. However, I was not allowed to watch the television or use my cell phone. Upon asking about my discharge date, he assured me that he would try to get me discharged as soon as possible, but he also cautioned that the decision would be made by the medical team. However, he mentioned that I was an obedient and disciplined patient, and he was positively expecting a rapid recovery for me. On this positive note, I went to sleep, dreaming about my home sweet home and my further plans to join the teaching work.

The next day, the entire team which was helping me in my treatment tried to get answers from me by presenting several questions on the same pattern that were asked the previous day. After collecting those answers, they discussed the outcome with my husband. They all were on the same point. They were positioning me either as the case of the memory loss or the hearing damage. They also expressed that I might be the case of the combination of both issues. My husband told the team that in the morning hours, I asked him about his job, busy schedule, and schoolwork, thus, my memory was functioning well. Finally, he was able to convince the team against the case of memory loss. To his relief, the team decided to conduct a hearing test, which would be formerly done with the medical aids and plans.

Since I could not walk even a few steps properly, I was taken to the hearing testing centre in a comfortable wheelchair. The nurse was excellent and polite who made me feel comfortable. We passed through many lobbies and then took an elevator. Finally, we landed in a room which was well equipped with the hearing test materials. There were several charts, pictures, and diagrams, which were posted on the walls.

Inside the testing room, one medical practitioner was carrying the test. On her instructions, I occupied a specially designed chair. A headset, an earphone and later plugs were connected to my ears properly. She asked some questions for half hour in repetitive manner, but later I could partially remember her questions. Then, she showed me the red and blue colour-waves like design on computer screen. She explained the internal ear system and conveyed me that my internal ear bones were damaged because of injury. Despite of her illustrative explanation, I could partially comprehend what she had said.

The members of the medical team, especially the social worker, told my husband to be with them to help them in monitoring the further progress. Thus, he could help them in making further decisions and chalking the roadmap of my treatment. On his side, he was still expecting me to get discharged in a couple of days. He was counting on the words of the radiologist, who told him that the head injury was not worsening anymore, and it would get automatically healed. The doctor was correct, but he had also mentioned that the date of discharge would be decided by the entire medical team after discussing all test results. Thus, on the wheelchair, and along with a nurse, I returned to my room. By hanging with the delicate thread of mental strength, I was swinging between the hope and the despair. Moreover, I was considerably tired after having the long session of questioning followed by almost half an hour of hearing testing. Thus, I was relieved when the nurse gave me medicine and I slept for a couple of hours.

I woke up around in the evening. My husband was still there reading a book. My mind was relatively clear after the nap, so I asked him about my chances of getting discharged and returning to home. He mentioned that since the injury was almost recovered, and there was no memory loss, the medical team would not tell me to stay in the hospital, just for having some hearing problem. He also mentioned that the experienced nurses of the ward had the same positive opinion. I had no idea how long we talked on this topic. He almost assured me that we would be in our home soon. His assurance helped me in regaining the peace of mind. He was still on the chair, when I went to sleep after having the night medicine dose from the nurse. I had an undisturbed sleep, not because of my clear mind, but because of the last night's medical dose, which was highly effective. My diet was almost stable, though the food was still tasteless for me. I was consuming small amount of meal four times, and therefore getting regular energy supply. Consequently, my body started functioning well and the medicines had the desired impact on my mind.

In tough time, we recall pleasant memories from our childhood. At least, I do the same. Despite of my husband's assurance, my mind was shadowed by unclear doubts about my health recovery. That shadow made me nostalgic, and I found a slight change in my thinking pattern. I started recalling my elder sister, Sagira Appi. In my childhood, she would sit beside my bed whenever I would fall sick. Now, I wished her to be on my bed side, caress my head, and pray for my quick recovery.

I knew after the hearing test that there was a big hearing loss. Obviously, the doctors were about to give me related required instructions. Therefore, my stay period in the hospital could be extended. I had been always living an active life, so now all the sudden remaining bed ridden was an unbearable torture for me. To reduce my worries, I was aimlessly asking questions to my husband about the further treatment course. As expected, he was painting a positive picture, though he did not know himself what was coming next.

After lunch, the medical team concluded that there was no cognitive issue. My wrong answers were related to the hearing loss. The team's words and approach bolstered my courage and confidence. However, a permanent damage to the body was a shock for me. Therefore, when I came out of the medical team cabin, I was in the silent mode ignoring everyone including my husband. I did not need to talk to him immediately, because he would never ask questions to me about my treatment. The medical team was providing him with the firsthand information.

Normally, my husband plays the role of a speaker, and I remain the listener. However, that day I decided to be a speaker. However, I could not discuss with him about the worries on my mind. Rather, to initiate a discussion, I turned nostalgic, and narrated him most of the incidents from the New York visit, especially about the Statue of Liberty, which was my dream destination since I was a child. When I was studying in grade four, I saw a picture of the Statue of Liberty, and asked my father if we could visit there. On that my father laughed and explained that it was in the United State of America, which was far away. I childishly expressed my determination to visit there in future. While narrating all these pieces of memory collection to my husband, I went back into the dream trip with my open eyes. I started visualising my active days when I would move fast while enjoying the tours. That visualisation started giving me the strength. However, as soon as I saw the nurse approaching towards me with the medicines, I came back to the bitter reality. After the departure of the nurse, I kept chatting with my husband that brought me to my sleeping time. Once again, I was on my comfortable bed with the closed eyes but with several questions that might remain unanswered till the next morning.

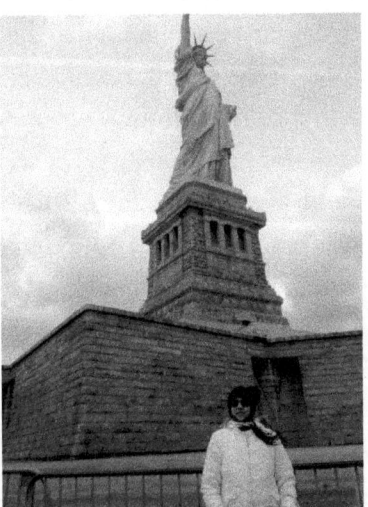

Statue of Liberty: My Dream

The stress of the damaged ear gave me the disturbed sleep. In my mind, the cardinal question was - if I would be able to go back to my usual active lifestyle. I came out of the circles of my thoughts when the nurse came to sponge me. Later, she gave me the morning dose of the medicine. I must mention here that all the nurses on my room duty, either on the day or the night shifts, were extremely professional, courteous, compassionate and understanding. They never made me feel that I was a liability for them despite of having many other responsibilities on their shoulders. They would try to make me feel at home by asking questions about my family life and would tell about their family lives.

While lying on my bed, I would frequently think about my past. I recalled my previous falls. In childhood, a cow hit me when I was about to go to attend a friend's birthday. My clothes were torn, and I was crying. My mother got me dressed again with the instructions to be careful. The next memorable fall was in the educational training days. A vehicle approached nearby abruptly that made me collapsed on the road and I was hurt. My classmates carried me to the home. Then, I had a fall in the school where I was working, while participating in a game. My both knees were badly hurt but I was not hospitalised. However, all those "falls" occurred years ago and were like a distant past for me. Nonetheless as they say, the past keeps haunting you. The same was true in my case.

My chain of nostalgic thoughts was broken by my husband's entry who brought some homemade food and clothing for me. He mentioned that the hospital staff was expressing positive assumptions about my recovery, and I would soon get discharged. I could not decide how to react, as the date of discharge was appearing elusive to me. They were collecting comprehensive information on my hearing and cognitive capabilities. They were also seeking more details from the hearing analysis expert and the radiologist. After all, they had the biggest say in making the decision. The medical side of the team was maintaining that the brain was functioning fine and would be on the path of improvement as my body would regain the strength. However, the speech therapist and the social worker would keep expressing that I was an actively working lady who must go back to the workforce after regaining the previous capabilities and skills, and that process must be completed under the supervision of the experts and authorities.

The next day, while eating my breakfast my husband was providing me updates on my son's studies. As usual, he brought some home cooked food and clothes. After the lunch, the medical team arrived on the scene. As usual, they had some testing questions, related to my personal information and my professional knowledge. My husband was helping me in understanding the questions, so it was relatively easy for me to comprehend and reply those questions. However, working on picture sheets was neither easy nor fluent task for me. I would feel fatigued after answering only two or three questions. Nonetheless, to my surprise, the team got somewhat impressed with my moderately improved performance. All the team members expressed that that there were limited but significant signs of improvements.

Finding me tired, they asked if I wanted to sleep. However, I declined, so they started discussing with my husband about the plan of my probable discharge, which was not finalised yet. They mentioned that I would be monitored at home all the time as one trained attendant would be given to assist and guide me. They had also mentioned that my husband needed to remain available all the time at home even when I was sleeping. Since my husband knew that my son was about to return home after his exams, my husband assured the team that someone would be always at home to look after me.

Further, the team members asked the details about my son. They mentioned that someone on the behalf of the hospital would contact him to provide him with the updates on my probable discharge and to get confirmation about his availability. One of them mentioned that the hospital had an encouraging observation about our family members, as the radiologist had already interacted with my son. Thus, such positive reports were prompting them to lean towards the idea of my discharge.

The team further mentioned that given my physical and mental conditions, I must get all required facilities on the ground floor. Thus, I should not use the stairs to complete any task. The team also added that the family members must also stay with me on the ground floor.

They also added that the hospital would like to inspect my house before granting me the discharge. My husband explained that the kitchen, the washroom, and the living room were located on the ground floor. Even though we had two bedrooms, the computer room, and another washroom on the upper floor, it was not needed to go upstairs for any reason. The first floor could be modified to make all the arrangements. He also explained that my son had a study room in the basement, and a television was also placed there. The team insisted that I must avoid the television for at least one month. I thought that following all these conditions was a tough exercise but not a bad proposition if I could go home.

The team members further explained that the home atmosphere would help me in getting recovered quite quickly. Thus, to keep me in the familiar environment of the home, the hospital could allow my early discharge. They also added that the hospital staff had found me a disciplined patient, having a cooperative family. However, they also mentioned that there were other factors, like additional medical tests and reports that would determine my further treatment plan and discharge date. That was the longest period that the team had spent with me. Fortunately, my husband was there to respond all the questions. Perhaps, the team had scheduled the discussion perceiving his availability. I was quite delighted to know that I was on the way of getting discharged. During the entire evening, I discussed with my husband about the further arrangements that we needed to make at home after my discharge. Meantime I had my dinner and medications also. However, we kept chatting all the time, and I did not know when I went to sleep.

The next day, the social worker visited. An unpleasant information was written on her face. She had an extensive talk with me, and then with my husband to collect some significant details. Then, she told me that only having rest at home environment would not help me. To get recovered completely, I needed the medical observation, the psychological support, the educational guidance, the nutritional input, and some specific physio exercises monitored by the experts. She politely urged me to utilise all those facilities provided by the system. She assured me that she would certainly recommend for my discharge. However, she cautioned that I should not remain adamant for leaving the hospital in hurry, if the medical team decided me to stay. She added that under the experts' observation, I would be in the better position of getting the fast recovery. She left the room, unintentionally putting me and my husband in the pool of contemplation. After discussing with my husband, I decided to go for the extended stay in the hospital. It was the late night, so I closed my moist eyes, expecting for the best.

When I woke up the next day, I was feeling a bit sad because I had to stay in hospital longer than expected. However, that negative reaction was my momentary laid-back attitude and not the permanent disappointment or rejection. I knew that there was much more remaining for me in the future, if I got recovered. After lunch, the social worker came to covey us that the next day, I was going to be shifted to the Parkwood Hospital for rehabilitation in the Acquired Brain Injury Inpatient Program. The Parkwood Hospital was close to the Victoria Hospital, just across the road. She explained that the monitoring team, having all sorts of experts in it, had decided to shift me for certain reasons. At first, there was no more possibility of my brain injury getting worsened. Then, I needed a different process for treatment that could be available at the Parkwood. Moreover, I would be brought back on the regular basis to the Victoria from the Parkwood for required check ups. She expressed her good wishes and delivered many other kind words, as the nice lady she was. Therefore, with her explanation, I realised that my brain injury was healing on its own. However, monitoring its healing process at the Parkwood was the matter of the teamwork. The team would have several medical experts and non-medical therapists. They all would observe the negative impact of the brain injury on my physical and mental capabilities. They would also support me in getting back those capabilities. Even though the medical experts would monitor the healing process, no single expert would be the authority in making the final decision for the entire case, like shifting me temporarily out of the Parkwood, if needed, for a different treatment.

CHAPTER 2

THE REHABILITATION AT PARKWOOD

"A rehabilitation that brings gradual and slow improvements may be frustrating, but it is safe. All quickly affecting things, be it a rehabilitation, a medicine, or a personality, are mostly unsafe."

Thursday, April 19, 2018

DURING THE BREAKFAST, a doctor entered the room and asked, "Firoza, how are you feeling?" I was happy to hear my name after a long time. She informed me that I would be moved to the Parkwood at 10:00 am. Perhaps, she read anxiety over my face, thus she assured me that I would be fine. She further explained that I needed several occupational and physiotherapist lessons to regain my professional capabilities. She added that after the ten-day treatment at the Victoria, I was stabilized but still I needed to spend more time with the rehabilitation hospital that would help me in learning to perform the basic professional tasks. I thanked her for her help.

I was shifted to Parkwood on Thursday, April 19, 2018. The nurse helped me in collecting my belongings before 10 am. Meantime, two hospital attendants appeared, introduced themselves, and brought a stretcher. They carried me in the stretcher to the elevator. While moving out, I thanked to everyone around me from the hospital staff and wished them good luck. At Parkwood, the assistants helped me in approaching at the reception. Despite of all my efforts, I was unable to stand on my own. However, I needed to be stable at the reception, so I was standing with the support of the wall. Once the formality was completed at the reception, two attendants brought me in the stretcher to the bed in the room 155 of the Block A. I thanked them before they left.

Soon, a nurse entered the room. After the formal introduction, she gave me two tablets of Tylenol for coping with the headache. This was not a major issue and it had nothing do with my traumatic brain injury. The tablets were quick at making their impact and I slept very soon. Soon, Dr. Alam visited me. He knew our family since 2009. His wife, Sameena, was my close friend. Considering my weak mental condition, Dr. Alam introduced himself. Still, I could not recall him. To ignite my memory, he asked about my family. I told him that my husband was about to arrive at the Parkwood, and my son was in Waterloo. He shook his head, read my information, and made some suggestions, before leaving. I felt embarrassed as I recognised him after his departure. However, his presence in the hospital was reassuring for me.

After half hour, a social worker Sarah Carroll, from the Parkwood, entered the room. She had all the information on my case, as her counterpart from the Victoria updated her. After the formal introduction, she told me that she was the in-charge of my workplace injury case. After her departure, my husband came. He had brought food and other things for me. We were talking on general topics related to our home when Dr. Alam revisited. Since they both knew each other well, they started talking. However, before leaving, he sympathetically told my husband that he was not expecting us to meet in those circumstances. Finally, he assured us that everything would be fine after some time.

My husband stayed there till 4 pm and then left. Shortly, a physiotherapist came with the nurse with a rollator walker. It was a shock for me. I jumped to the conclusion that I had to remain in the walker for the rest of my life. I had never used rollator walker before but had seen many disabled persons using walkers. I thought that the permanent disability doubt, which was hovering over my head from the last two days, had turned into the reality. That thought made me tearful. However, for my relief, the physiotherapist explained that the walker was for my temporary support. She further added that I could not afford to lose my balance, thus I must use the rollator walker while moving. I shook my head in confirmation.

I was observing the walker, when the nurse came, showed me the menu, and asked about my meal choices. I selected the vegetarian food. However, I knew that my selection would not make me to eat much. Having consumed the meal in the Victoria for ten days, I could say that the food would be healthful but tasteless for me. Moreover, I had lost most of my appetite. My husband reappeared with my personal things that I asked for. My husband updated me on our home and related matters. We chatted for a while, but he needed to leave by the end of the visiting hours. Before sleeping, I asked for a warm blanket, which the nurse brought. I closed my eyes and tried to sleep in the new place. I knew that it was not an easy task.

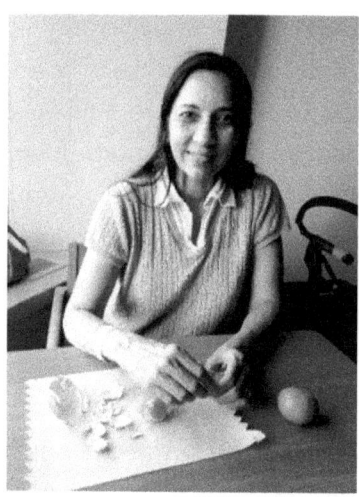

At Parkwood

From next day, my rehabilitation at Parkwood started. When I woke up, a nurse brought a medical cart, which was a common medical device for a long-term patient. Since it was a novel and unfamiliar equipment for me, I got surprised. She looked at my record, which was fed in the computer attached to the cart. Then, she gave me two tablets and one needle for probably regaining the strength because soon I felt relatively rejuvenated. She told me that I was scheduled to visit the Western University hospital after the lunch. She also assured that an assistant would be provided to support me. Travelling from Parkwood to Western university was time consuming, because of the busy traffic of the city during the noon hours.

After looking at my appointment, the reception informed me that I was being checked by the Oral maxillofacial Service at the University Hospital. The medical team would observe my face and neck using CT scan for finding any suspected fracture because of the accident. I was guided towards the doctor's room. Two student doctors were also there. They asked me some basic questions, and then told me to narrate the accident details. I guessed that they were instructed to find out if I had any facial or neck injury because of the fall on the stairs. I narrated whatever I could recall. Shortly, the doctor entered the room and after asking some formal questions, he inspected my neck and my jaws. He did some more check ups and then declared that I had no fractures on my facial bones. When I came back to Parkwood, Dr. Alam did the routine check ups and asked some questions. I was feeling dizzy, so had some rest when he left the room. Then my husband came with some home cooked food and fruits. I ate some amount of soft food. He left when the period of visiting hours finished as we were strictly following the visiting hours' rules. Finally, I slept relatively with ease as I was tired and exhausted.

When I woke up the next day, I was greeted by a nurse. She was very friendly and made sure that I was feeling comfortable. She gave me my prescribed medicines. Later, a physiotherapist came and gave me walking practice with the help of rollator walker. The practice was not strenuous, but I felt tired after doing some walking. The physiotherapist realized my exhaustion and told me to have some rest. I had a short nap till the visiting hours began. My husband arrived soon and told me that my son was visiting during the weekend. I was very excited to meet my son.

Dr. Alam came for the regular check up. He talked to my husband for a while and told me that I was recovering well. He said that in the case of traumatic brain injury, a patient would quickly get recovered at the initial stage, but later improvements might happen slowly. I felt comfortable for having a familiar doctor around to convey me the facts. Sameena, Dr. Alam's wife and my close friend, arrived. It felt good to talk to her as after long time I was talking to any of my friends.

The next day, my son visited me along with my husband. I was very happy to see him. I missed talking to my son. He was also very happy to see me. Before my accident, we used to spend a lot of time together. I was glad that I had the much-needed family support with me.

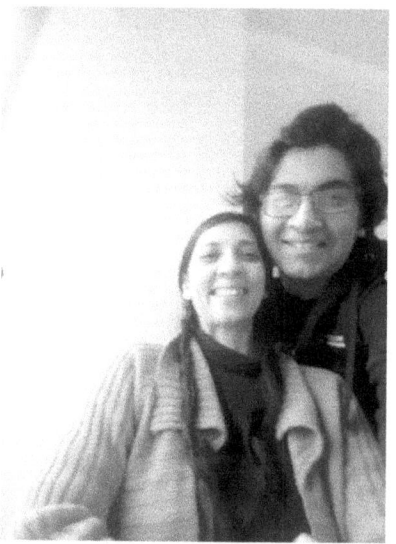

With My Son at Parkwood

Next day, the occupational therapist Jillian Kuepfer arrived on the scheduled time. We had greetings and the formal introduction. Then, she told me that her job was to find out the level of professional skill I possess, and the course of improvement, if needed, to enhance the level of those professional skills as per my job requirements. She gave me some basic math calculations. I tried to focus on them, but my several answers went wrong. I could not figure out why I did those mistakes despites of being a math teacher. However, the therapist encouraged me stating that such silly mistakes could appear after having the accident shock. I was deeply tired after finishing the occupational therapy lesson. I felt that it was extremely lengthy, though it was only half an hour long. She left after encouraging me with some nice comments and I rested on the bed.

However, I knew that as per the timetable, the physiotherapist would come. As expected, she came on her scheduled time. Her name was Mellissa Fielding. She took me to a small gym. She brought a blue coloured soft balanced board for me. Before instructing me to do an activity, she demonstrated how to stand on the balance board. On my turn, I tried to repeat what she had demonstrated. I noticed that I was not steady though she was patiently supporting me. I tried three times, and the last two efforts were relatively better, though not perfect.

As the visiting hours began, my son, Sharon, came. I was happy and excited to tell him about the therapy lessons. I had trouble in speaking in flow, thus I slowly explained about the rollator walker and other equipment I used in the gym. It was the dinner time and we ate together. Mostly, I ate home-made food along with some hospital food. The chatting with my son was soothing. It rapidly brought me to my sleeping time. Once again, I was on my comfortable bed with the closed eyes.

Next day, I had appointment with Laura Hanley, occupational therapist. She took me in the same small gym. She gave me a sheet, showing two pictures having some differences and similarities. My task was to find out similarities in those two pictures. She hinted that there might be around ten similarities, but I could find only four. She encouraged me even after my low performance. She said that such activities would help me in boosting my cognitive skills. Then she gave me a maths sheet for doing basic math calculations. I was confident for doing it well for being a math teacher. It took me longer time to complete, but I did it correctly. Thereby, the lessons were over, so she brought me to my room. After saying some inspiring words, she left. After lunch, Dr. Alam visited and asked general questions. When I told him that sometimes I felt dizzy, hence avoid eating, he approved my decision, mentioning that vomiting was the most dangerous factor in a brain injury case. After performing his regular check up and taking some notes, he left. Then, Sharon, my son, came on the commencement of the visiting hours. He brought home cooked food and some fruits too. I ate oranges and talked with him on several topics. He left when the visiting hours finished.

When he left, I started recalling my son's phone calls when I would be in the school for work in India. He was too young to stay alone after his school hours, so he stayed with my friend, Vandana Mojhariya's home for almost one hour. She was very kind-hearted lady. He would stay with her in her home which was nearby the school. However, he would find his few after school hours too long and would make calls to me in his cute voice. Those pieces of memories brought a smile on my lips. I was happy that my son would be there the next day.

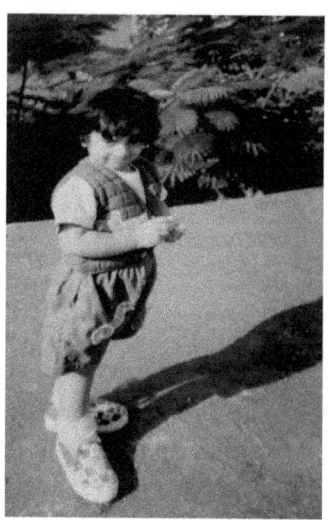

My cute son as a baby

When I woke up, I was greeted by my nurse. She was very friendly and gave me my prescribed medication. I had to attend a session of occupational therapist, which was similar to the previous session. Later, I had an appointment with Sarah McLean, the physiotherapist assistant. She took me to the physiotherapy room. She told me to perform one leg standing act on the balance board. I tried to remain in the standing position without taking any support of rollator walker but lost my balance. Sarah encouraged me and told me not to lose hope.

Soon, I had lunch at my regular time. After having lunch, I took a short nap. Dr Alam came on his scheduled time for the routine check up and expressed his satisfaction about my improvement. I narrated what activities I had done during the last three hours, and the associated difficulties that I faced. He listened everything patiently and explained that such difficulties would keep surfacing. He suggested to follow the instructions given by the nurses, the physiotherapist and the occupational therapist to overcome those difficulties.

After Dr. Alam left, I was resting on the bed waiting for my son. My son came right on time and he was chatting with me like a chatterbox. He took my pictures while I was peeling oranges. I didn't know how fast the time flew by. Soon, the visiting hours were over and my son was leaving. He tucked me in bed and wrapped a blanket around me before leaving. I slept very peacefully because I got to spend some quality moments with my son.

Next morning, during my session with the occupational therapist, she gave me the task of matching the pictures with the given statements. It was a subjective task, having no definite answers, but I completed the task well. Then, she showed me some memory games. One of them was recalling the articles. She would show some articles for thirty seconds and then would hide them. I had to recall the seen articles. I did well on this assignment too. After my session was over, I had training session with the physiotherapist. We went to the gym, where she gave me a new task of collecting pilons. She would keep pilons in the different sections of the room and I had to collect them in a line. She gave me that exercise two times. On some occasions, I was about to lose my balance, but she was always behind me to keep me in the balance.

Dr. Alam came on his scheduled time and asked questions about my all step exercises, which I performed that day. I narrated the whole session and then told him that I was feeling tired. He asked about my son as he knew him well. After completing his routine check up, he left. In the visiting hours my son came and brought six oranges and some homemade food. To entertain me, he was playing songs on his phone. However, I could not follow them though the sound was loud. As per my schedule, the hospital served the dinner, but I ate only the homemade food. I told my son to eat all cheese food catered by the hospital. He ate it readily, though he would also prefer the spicy food. After that, instead of playing the cards, we had a long-elaborated chatting till the end of the visiting hours. Before leaving, he covered me with the blanket on my request.

Next day, the nurse informed me that my room was scheduled to be changed after breakfast. Another change for my schedule was that instead of two scheduled classes, occupational therapy and physiotherapy, now I had four classes to attend. In the physio class both Sarah, the assistant, and Melissa, the physio were present. They gave me balance balloon kicking practice. It was appearing easy in the beginning, but I found it difficult while doing it. They gave me five minutes to do it. Then, I did a thirty-step exercise on the balance board without having a support. Soon, it was my time for lunch. I was slowly adjusting to the food provided by the hospital. I took my routine nap after my lunch to take some rest and get refreshed ahead of more classes. Dr. Alam came soon after I woke up for his regular check up. He was happy with my progress. After his check up, Sarah, the assistant physio came. In this class, I had to catch the ball while standing on a cushion. It was hard to keep the balance, but I performed without losing my stability. Sarah expressed that she was satisfied with my performance. Her assuring words and the improved performance enhanced my confidence, giving me a substantial hope of returning the home. Soon, my son came in the visiting hours. He brought the playing cards with him. We played some games and I won a few of them. Even though they were only cards games, it gave me belief that I was on the right track for recovery.

As per the Parkwood schedule, there were no therapy classes during the weekend. Even though the regular classes would flow with the slow pace, I would get tired. Thus, on the weekends I had an opportunity to relax. While I was sitting by my room's window, I was a group of ducklings with their parents. They were swimming in a nearby pond. I found this parental guidance and its impact on the ducklings quite amusing. It reminded me how I used to treat my son, when he was a toddler.

Watching the parents protecting the ducklings, I recalled an incident, when a hen attacked me in my childhood. I was just five-year-old at that time. A hen was watching her young chicks as they were eating and playing. The chicks were soft, bright and cute. I could not prevent myself from touching them. Seeing that I was trying to hold the chicks in my hands, the hen mistakenly concluded that I was trying to harm them. She jumped on me and I collapsed on the ground losing my balance. Then my mother came, consoled me explaining that the hen had to protect her chicks, and got me prepared for the school.

My husband and son came to visit me during the visiting hours. We enjoyed the home cooked food and played cards games. Once again I managed to win a few games and I was enjoying my success. For a few moments, I felt like I had not been affected by the accident at all. By the end of the visiting hours, I gave my son a greeting card that I had prepared. Earlier, I used to give him a small amount of money as token of blessings at the beginning of every semester. Nevertheless, at that moment, I felt that my hand made card would make more sense. In addition, I gave him three toonies that was all I had that time. He has still those coins and the card with him. He carries them as my blessings. He hugged me before leaving. It was very emotional moment for me, but I hid my tears.

Next morning, I had to take shower as per my schedule. I was hesitating as it was my first shower in the hospital. There was no tub in my washroom. The nurses would give me the sponging. I needed to keep my clothing prepared to change the outfits after having the sponging. However, now I had the opportunity of taking proper shower though on my own. The shower was followed by the breakfast. Then, Jillian, the occupational therapist, came. She took me to her therapy room. I noticed that the physiotherapist and occupational therapist both were sharing the room for delivering their therapy lessons. She gave me some worksheets for practice to help me in developing my cognitive skills. The next was physiotherapy class with Sarah, the assistant physiotherapist. On the soft balance board, she gave me the step practice. After that she put me on the stand bicycle and told me to paddle slowly. The next exercise was to repeat thirty steps on a balance board. It was tiring but I did it without asking for a support. After lunch, Dr. Mackenzie and Dr. Alam came. Dr Mackenzie came to see me for the first time. I noticed that she was pregnant but still she was active. She checked my knees by tapping them with a small soft tool to find out whether my involuntary reflexes were functioning. She was satisfied with the outcome and said that I was recovering well.

I took a nap after the doctors' departure. Then, the assistant occupational therapist came, with the head therapist, Jillian. They gave me some worksheets for testing my cognitive skills. Also, they asked about the time I had spent with my family. Subsequently, they gave me an exercise of circling the objects on the sale. I used my glasses for completing the exercise. After checking my work, they said that I did well on all the given assignments. Then, I got the homework sheet. They told me that I would get regular homework related to math and language. They further explained that in math, I would get both, simple calculations and reasoning questions. They added that in language, I would mostly get the exercises based on the passage reading. Noticing my concern, they assured that there would be no time limit for solving any worksheet.

I noticed that in my all classes the instructors were trying to mix regular exercises with personal chatting, perhaps to check my social interest and desire for the social connection. Although they had extended my class hours, they would closely watch my energy level and would provide me breaks whenever needed. I was grateful for their compassionate and caring approach.

May, 2018

On May 1, I had my medical appointment scheduled 11 am. After having the medication and the breakfast, I had free time, so I got engaged in making notes for my diary. Since, I overheard two visitors discussing about their trip to the South America, I started jotting notes on my trip to the United States with my son.

After finishing his bachelor's degree, he planned to go on a tour across the western part of the United Sates. He wanted to visit New Orleans, San Diego, San Francisco, and Chicago. My husband, who would still consider him a child and was unable to join him because of his professional commitments, told me to go with him to ensure his safety. We visited many enjoyable spots. My son thanked me for being with him otherwise he would have missed places like the Golden Gate Bridge. The train journey was scenic, covering several mountains, rivers, and towns. I would get up in the morning and would occupy a seat in the observation deck. My son would bring food, mostly fruits, for me. His managing abilities convinced me that he was no more a child and now he was an independent and mature person. That realisation was the greatest finding of the tour.

When we were in Chicago, we visited the Willis Tower, formerly known as Sears Tower. It was once the tallest building in the North America. There was an observation deck at the top of the building, from where the whole city could be seen. The observation deck was completely made of the glass. Its floor was also made of the glass, so standing in the deck would feel like standing in the sky. I was extremely excited for going in the observation deck. However, my son was feeling a bit nervous as he feared heights. Thinking about his nervousness, made me compare my current condition to my old self. At present, I could not even imagine about standing near the stairs. This made me appreciate my past experiences even more.

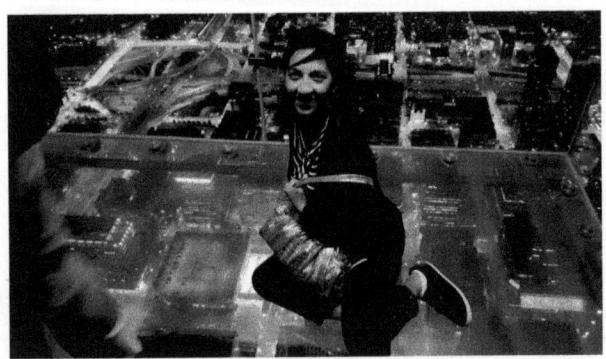

Not Afraid of Heights: At Willis Tower in Chicago

I put back the diary in my purse and started getting prepared for my appointment with a general neurosurgeon. While I was waiting for the neurosurgeon, I chatted with the assistant. She told me that she would work on many other supporting activities. I felt relaxed because of her easy-going personality. She asked about my profession, family and background. I happily shared many details with her. After long time, I was sitting and chatting in a non-hospital atmosphere which was appearing to me more like an airport lounge though it was still a hospital. The neurosurgeon came on her scheduled time. She was familiar to me, as I had seen her in the Victoria Hospital too during my initial check ups. She asked about my hearing problems. I mentioned that my hearing check up appointment was scheduled on May 3 at the Western University hospital. She told me that I was appearing much better than before. She also asked about my husband, as she had a discussion with him during my initial check ups. To my relief, she just conversed with me and did not perform any check-up. When I came back from my appointment, I had a class with physio. She gave me practice on the balance board and told me to do some exercises on the medicine ball. I could not do well in both activities because I was tired. After the class, I did homework for the next half hour. I did math exercises well but started feeling dizzy, so I took a break. Then, the occupational therapist came, and we went in the therapy room. She gave me exercise for practicing my cognitive skills. She checked my sheets and found them mostly correct. We came back to my room after and I decided to sleep early as I was exhausted.

Next day, I had again four scheduled classes, so I was busy all day. On the instructions of the occupational therapist, I tried to write on a blackboard, but my writing was not straight. I got horrified for not performing the basic task of a teacher. Prior to the accident, I would write well on a board. Laura was observing from the outside. She assured that I did good on the blackboard writing assignment, though I knew I did not. On my next assignment, another assistant therapist and a student therapist gave me a binder to write my schedule. I was glad that according to the schedule, I would get shower on alternate days. Then, Sarah, the social worker, asked me whether I would participate in the Acquired Brain Injury Unmasking Painting event, which was scheduled on the next day. I told her that I would be very happy to participate in the event.

Melissa, the physiotherapist, gave me a new task - balancing on a foam cushion and catching the thrown balls. Since balancing the body was still a challenge for me, I could not perform the task well. I relaxed for a while and then started a new task, balance board walking with hand coordination. I performed it moderately well. The lunch break brought the much-needed relief for me. I was wondering that balancing the body was still an unresolved question for me though all therapists were trying to help me on that issue. After lunch, Dr Alam visited and asked me about my general well-being. Finding me a little uneasy, he asked if I had headache. I told him that I was only a little tired. He left after delivering some consoling words.

Connie Ferri, speech therapist provided me an amplifier for assisting in hearing. She had explained its operation method. Thus, I could hear relatively clearly, but still I could not understand everything. This device was very helpful when I was listening to the instructions during the Acquired Brain Injury Unmasking Painting event. Some patients used oil paint. However, I used colour pencils because I did not want to create mess. I got a sheet to depict my experience about the brain injury. I drew and decorated a mask and put a quotation mark on it, with the caption - Hope is the Way of Life; Be Calm. While working, I talked to other patients. It was appearing like working in an art class. The organisers took our pictures and asked for permission to publish them in the media.

I wrote:

Firoza's mask

The Cause of the Brain Injury: On Monday, April 09, 2018 at 11:35 - 40 am, I fell from Montcalm Secondary School's second floor stairs and I got a brain injury.

The Explanation of the Mask: My mask reflects how I felt after suffering from the brain injury. After one week, I understood that I must improve by rehab. I was brought to the Parkwood Institute. The Parkwood team gives me everyday therapy to improve my body coordination and brain work. The Parkwood team is very cooperative. I know that my brain injury will now be a challenge for me. However, I believe that if I keep patience and calm, I can improve. Still, I am joyful, courageous, and proud of myself. I am also blessed because I got the Parkwood Institute team to support me in various ways so I can improve my brain functioning again.

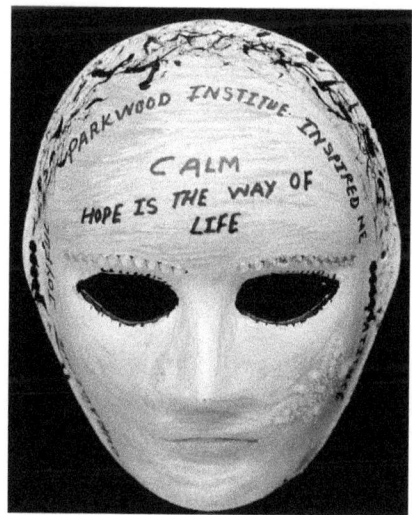

My Brain Mask

I had a sense of content for participating in a creative activity. I went to the bed, recalling my school-working days when I would prepare artwork for school function. In that act of recalling, I fell asleep in deep sleep.

Next day, I had my hearing check up appointment at the Western University hospital with Dr. Parnes. After arriving in the doctor's cabin and upon asking, I narrated the details about the accident to Dr Parnes and a student doctor. The doctor asked some more questions about my brain injury and made some notes based on my replies. He encouraged me to continue my all efforts and praised me for my nerves. He checked my ears and did not find any new problem. However, he said that he would keep observing my ears in the regular intervals. He gave me the next appointment after one month. When I came back to Parkwood, Stephanie Muir, the speech therapist, allowed me for the late therapy session. She gave me a booklet to complete. Meanwhile, she asked me about my ear checkup appointment. I narrated all about the meeting with Dr Parnes. She had some papers with her. After reading them carefully, she told me that I would get discharged on May 31.

Although it was a great piece of information, I had a sort of mixed reaction. On one hand, I was glad to know the fixed date of the discharge. However, on the other hand, I felt low to know that I had to stay in the Parkwood for the entire month. Soon, Dr. Alam came for the check up. He was satisfied with the progress. He said that I was allowed by the medical team supervising me to stay at the home on the weekends. Afterwards, the social worker, Sarah, also confirmed my home staying during the weekends, cautioning that I needed to be careful as I was still under the medical observation.

When my son arrived, I showed him enthusiastically my walk without using the walker support. I brought my dinner tray by myself and put it on the shelf without any help too. It was the first time after my accident that I handled my food tray by myself. I was excited like a toddler who had just learned to walk and wanted to surprise others by displaying it. Later, I also told him about the permission I got for my home visits on weekends. He was excited for seeing me at home. I reminded him that he needed to be at 7:30 am at hospital to pick me. He assured that he would be there on time. Then, we played cards for a while. We stopped playing when I felt tired. We started chatting. I was so excited to see my home after a month. Before he left, I reminded him again to come on time. He reassured me and covered me by the blanket before leaving.

Next morning, I woke up early as I was excited to be back at my home. My son came on the right time. I was in the washroom as he was a little early. The nurse gave me the needle and the medication. She reminded me to follow all instructions about the diet, physiotherapy, walking, etc.

When I boarded in the car, I felt relaxed for being in a familiar vehicle with a familiar person after a long time - enormously lengthy period. I had been travelling in the ambulances and the taxis for almost a month with the professionals - drivers, nurses, assistants and other social workers. Although, they all were extremely caring and compassionate, I had still the feeling of being with the strangers in the strange vehicles, making me feel like I was a stranger for myself. During the entire drive, I wanted to walk in the open and fresh air. Indeed, I was excited for being in my son's car and was enjoying the drive. However, my preference had been always the long walks and not the long drives.

When I arrived at home, my son gave me the key to open the door. I was feeling that I got back the ownership of my home. In the front room, I rested myself in the sofa for a while. My husband had prepared the food for us and left in the fridge. My son brought the breakfast for me, keeping the kitchen clean and well arranged. We ate together, and he washed all the dishes. Since I was not allowed to go the upstairs alone where my bedroom was, he sat with me in the front room. He was watching a cricket game on the television, while I was resting. Later he provided me update of cricket match.

In the hospital, I could not observe my face in a mirror leisurely and clinically. I would be always supported by the nurses and the assistants. It would appear inappropriate to me to request them to wait for me till I observe my face thoroughly. However, I had a sense of concern if the accident had partially or temporarily damaged my face. I got relieved for finding none of such signs. My face was the same as it was before the accident, though the weakness was reflecting on it clearly. I recalled that on the day of the accident, I was getting prepared in front of the mirror. That was the last time when I had seen myself meticulously in a mirror. Also, that was the last day when I worked in the kitchen.

My husband came back from the work after a couple of hours. I hugged him. We all there had the lunch together. I took a brief nap as per the hospital instructions. Then, we played the cards for a while. I was sitting on the chair from where I could see the Wonderland road clearly. On my familiar seat, I felt that the time went fast. My husband had to go for the work at 6 pm. He reminded my son to drop me to the hospital on the right time. Meanwhile, my son helped me in overcoming the difficulties of the therapists' worksheet based on testing the cognitive skills. I completed my homework with his help.

Soon, it was my time to leave for the hospital. I was unwilling to leave my home but wanted to return to the hospital on the pre-determined time. I had the anticipation that the hospital will allow me to visit my home again if I follow the instructions meticulously. After arriving in the hospital, we informed the reception. Since I ate at the home, my son returned the dinner brought by the assistant. He left after I got settled in my room.

The last day's visit to my home made me wake up with the pleasant mind set. My son was coming to pick me up again. After arriving at the home, I went to my bedroom and had my lunch there. I kept watching through the window the movements of the traffic and the pedestrians on the Wonderland road. My son was sitting beside me and talking to me. Since, I was tired too, I had a nap. After waking up, I did the light exercises suggested by the physiotherapist while my son was studying. The time was flying, and soon it was time to go back to the hospital. However, I was not dejected or disillusioned now. I was happy about the time I had spent at my home. My son dropped me at the hospital. I had no phone, so I told him to inform my husband about my arrival in the hospital. I went to the bed as per the hospital rules, though I was not tired.

Next day, Sarah, the physiotherapist, took me the outdoors for the walk. It was the refreshing open-air activity that I always liked to do. The walkway was crisscross and would pass though the several beautiful settings, including the lush green grass, the dense olive bushes, the colourful flower plants, and the towering compressed trees. I was walking slowly and carefully but steadily. Sarah was happy with my walking as I had walked for an extended time covering a stretched distance after a long time. After our walk, I settled in the big lounge doing the homework. There were several buildings in front of the hospital, clearly visible from the lounge. Among all those setups, there was a daycare. Several kids would keep playing in the fenced yard.

That scenario made me recall my son playing with the toy train in his childhood, while I was working around. He would make his train with the LEGO blocks and would keep moving it on the different "tracks" in the home. Seeing his passion for the trains, sometimes, I would feel that he would be a train engineer in the future. In fact, he had developed an affinity for the trains in his early childhood, perhaps, because in India, he did railway tours since he was a toddler. We had visited several picnic spots and tourist places when he was still a child. His favourite activity was the cooking in the train pantry. He had consumed few delicious snacks from the train pantry during the several train journeys. Also, he had seen those kitchens from inside. Thus, he would pretend that he had prepared food and snacks in his pantry and would bring that food for me. I would pretend that I liked the food much and would pay him the fake money. He would be extremely happy with that act.

I had an appointment with the eye specialist doctor. She asked some questions about the accident to know if I had any problems related to the eye damage. Then, she showed me some familiar pictures of fruits and vegetables and told me to identify them mentioning their sizes and colours. After recording my answers, she did not take much time to conclude that there was no eye damage. However, she mentioned that I needed to do a follow check up with my optometrist.

Later, the assistant of the speech therapist guided me through the whole building. She showed me several sections, including the gym, the cafe, the library, the park, the spa room, and the shopping area. She told me to remember the locations of and the ways to all these areas as after some days I needed to go in all those places without a guide. Knowing my limited capabilities in recalling a new building set up, I was certain that I might make some mistakes while revisiting those sections. However, I tried to prepare a mental building map as accurately as possible. After that I came back to my room and took rest.

Next day, the assistant occupational therapist took me in the kitchen for preparing the lentil soup. We went by walk to an apartment, beautifully decorated and guarded by the security, who opened the door for us. The apartment was a home like setting, prepared for the patients who could not visit their homes. They would spend some hours there, so that they could feel that they were at their homes. The therapist brought me to the kitchen. She delivered some instructions, but I could not follow them completely as I was working without using the hearing amplifier. She told me to be careful about closing the stove as any mistake in that process might cause an accident. For completing the task, I prepared the lentil soup properly. However, I committed a mistake while closing the stove because I could not comprehend the given instructions for my hearing problem. I was not happy with myself that I made that mistake.

I returned to the recreation room after having the lunch. The rehabilitation therapist, April, joined me. She reminded me of another girl, also April by name, my son's friend, and now a PhD student. On April 9, the day of the accident, she was the only visitor in the emergency ward. Later, she visited to our new house too and spent a full day with us. She was a kind-hearted, intelligent and hardworking girl.

Next day, the occupational therapist led me again to the kitchen and gave an assignment of performing certain kitchen related tasks. She explained that it was a test of motor and cognitive skills. I used the microwave to prepare the hot water for making the tea and I served it to my therapists. Then, I had to complete another task, in which I had to circle the items, which were on the sale on a flyer. She was satisfied with my performance, though she said that I must work slowly to be careful. I was happy that I did not make the same mistakes again.

Later in the week, Karley, the assistant speech therapist, reminded me that I had to go for the memory test. She had shown me the building with all its areas and approaching ways. Now, I needed to recall all the routes and show her the entire building. I guided her correctly, from the elevator to the corner shop to the recreation hall etc. Finally, I brought her back to my room after showing all the sections. She was pleased by my performance and praised me for having a good memory. I was happy and confident for recalling everything correctly during the test.

While I was sitting in my room, I found some children playing hide and seek among the trees in the nearby daycare centre. That reminded me of my two siblings, Javed and Shamim, who were slightly older than me. We would play hide and seek at our home. Given the present confusion in mind about identities of simple things, I was surprised that it was easy in those childhood days to remember and recall who could hide where. It was perhaps possible because our child-world was limited, and other issues were not on our mind to make the life complex.

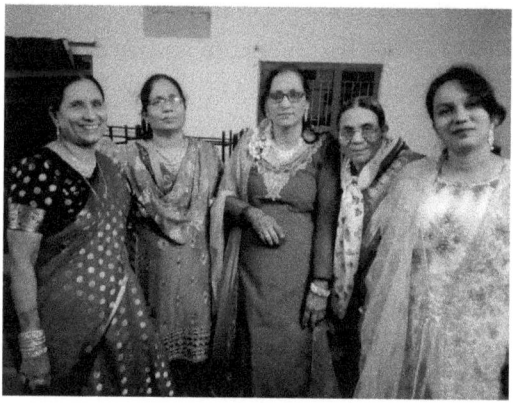

My Sisters

In the weekend, I woke up early and my son came on the right time to pick me up. While I was entering my home, I saw my neighbour's two cats; one was black and the other was white. They used to peep from the window whenever I would come out of my home. Sometimes, for the fun, I would show them my tongue. They would watch me standing still with curiosity. It would appear to me that they too started enjoying my presence around. We had become friends. I always had liking for pets. However, given our professional schedules, we did not have enough free time to keep pets. Nevertheless, I had close contact with two pets in my childhood days. The first was a calf, Jummi, which was given to our family by my oldest brother. The calf was lonely as his mother was living in a nearby village with my brother. We used to feed him milk by a bottle having a nipple on it. He would be extremely happy and exited whenever he would see us coming towards him with the bottle. He had developed a perfect understanding with us.

Another pet was a beautiful white cat having some black spots. She would live around our house. After some time, she bore four pretty kittens. We used to feed them with the food from our kitchen. We would enjoy the kittens playing around us. However, one night when the cat was sleeping with her kittens, another cat attacked her, and in that fight one kitten got killed. The cat was crying the whole night. We found out about the incident the next day. We were remorseful and sad, but the damage was done already. However, from that day we started taking extreme care of the cat and the kittens to ensure their safety.

My son brought breakfast and we ate together. Then, he started watching a cricket event on the television. For giving him the company, I was sitting beside him. During a commercial break, an advertisement showed the Taj Mahal, one of the seven wonders of the world. I started recalling my visit to the Taj Mahal in Agra, India. My son was only eight-year old then. My husband told him in the morning that he would get new shoes. We arrived at the Taj Mahal at noon, and the plan was to stay there till the late evening so that we could see that historical structure in the different shades of the sun and the moon – shining white, crimson orange, dusky blue and eventually milky cream. The place was full of the tourists. After viewing the Taj Mahal from inside and outside, we occupied a seat from where we could have the full view of the structure with its all four pillars, changing the shades. However, by evening, my son started turning impatient as he wanted to buy the new shoes. Although, my husband promised him to get shoes the next day if the market got closed early. Nevertheless, he did not listen to any logic or promise, and we had to head towards the market leaving the Taj Mahal, just after the sun setting. Thinking about the whole episode made me smile.

My husband came shortly and joined us. For the rest of day, I took rest and chatted with my family. Soon, it was my time to leave for the Parkwood. My husband cooked the food, said some encouraging words, and left for his work. I felt that the time flew away quickly. However, I was not disappointed or upset, because I was coming back tomorrow as well. My son dropped me to my room in the Parkwood and covered me with a warm blanket. I slept peacefully as I was excited to visit my home again the next day.

After coming home and eating breakfast, I did some physical exercises as prescribed by my physiotherapists. It made me tired, so I took some rest. My son was watching a cricket game on the television. My husband came back from the work around the lunch time. We all had the lunch together. After the lunch, I took some rest as the heavy lunch made me drowsy. I was joyfully perceiving that I was on a vacation and staying in a hotel as my family was doing everything for me. I was feeling like a special guest. After waking up, I played the cards with my son and husband. While playing, I saw that there were some kids playing hopscotch beside our home. I recalled my childhood days when I used to play hopscotch with my siblings, Javed, Salma and Shamim. Javed used to stop playing whenever he was about to lose. The kids who were playing in my neighbourhood, were also doing the same. It made me laugh as I liked using tricks for winning a game.

My husband left for his work. Soon, it was time for me to go back to the hospital. I was gloomy while leaving my home because the next five days I had to stay in the hospital. However, I was hopeful too for coming back again. I reminded myself that because of following all the medical instructions, I got opportunity to spend some quality time with my family, and if I kept continuing my disciplined practice, soon I would be permanently at the home. I wished my son good luck for his studies as he was leaving for Waterloo after dropping me at the hospital.

Next day, the physiotherapist asked me about the physical exercises I had done at the home. I explained that my son had supported me and demonstrated what I had done. She revised some exercises, and after adding some modifications, she told me to continue those revised exercises. Then, the occupational therapist visited and asked about my home visit experience. I related everything in the detail. For me, narrating the experience of the last four visits at home was like gaining the joy of visiting the home. Noticing my enthusiasm, she gave me a high five. I was in the state of a child who had recently found something new and unique and thus wanted to display it to others. In my last visit to the home, I had learned from my son how to solve trigonometry questions without using the tables or the charts. I explained the procedure to her. She was glad to learn it from me.

After that class, I settled in the small lobby with food. While eating reluctantly, I was looking at the garden beneath. It was simple yet spacious, having a vast open space for the daycare children's outdoor activities. Some kids, supervised by the adults, were playing there. The garden reminded me of my childhood picnic events that we would have in our neighbourhood garden. In my childhood, I would live in a colony designated for the employees of the Ballarpur Industries Limited, BILT. It was one of the most famous paper factories in India. My father was employed as a chartered accountant in BILT. Because of the industry, the town had a railway junction, having all major trains' stop. The town was well connected with the state transport bus services. Therefore, several schools, especially the elementary ones, even from the nearby district, would bring their students for the picnic in that beautiful and well-equipped garden. It had several plants and trees, slides, rides, and a merry-go-round. It was always fun to go in the colony garden as there were not many places of attraction for us in that town. In the garden, we would play the simple games, like cycling, chasing, hide and seek, and so on.

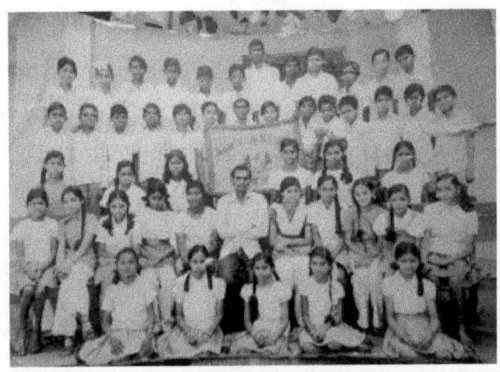

My childhood classmates

I came back to my room after finishing the lunch. Soon, Dr Alam and Dr Mackanzie, visited to perform their general check ups. They saw me standing nearby the room, so they approached me, asked few questions, and then from the next day allowed me to spend nights at home till my discharge. It was unexpected and delightful information for me. They had a meeting with other therapists and after completing my case assessment, they concluded to let me go to the home every night. However, I would need to visit the hospital every day for my therapy until my discharge. After some time, the nurse informed me that there would be no needle for me from that day. The needles were painful to some extent. I was pleased that I would have to take only limited medication. There was one more positive information for me. All therapists told me that soon I would be able to move as per my wish without taking the support of the walker, though I would need to keep the control on my physical movements. I recalled that I would do jumping, running, and many playful activities with my family before the accident. I might not be able to repeat those activities, but certainly I would not be moving around with the walker.

Next morning, there was a meeting with my medical team and the WSIB officials. The WSIB officials opened the meeting by expressing their sympathy and support in such dire situation for us. They also cleared that they would collect information from everyone present in the meeting, and then the final decision related to their office would be made. Sarah, in brief, stated my health condition after the accident, and mentioned that I had the substantial family support. The medical representative from the hospital read the report based on the assessments of my all regular supervising doctors. The report was long, but the bottom line was I had no life-threatening health issue, though I needed to be careful while moving around to avoid any further damage.

All the therapists read their final report. They all agreed that I had some cognitive issues because of the traumatic brain injury as well as hearing loss but overall, I was safe to leave the hospital. They said that I needed further support in all areas – physio, speech, recreation, and occupation – in order to get recovered completely. The WSIB officials summed up all the reports, stating that their office would provide all required support, and also assured that we could contact them at any point for seeking assistance and guidance.

Finally, at the meeting it was decided that I could go back to my home every day. However, I would need to visit the hospital to attend different therapies during the weekdays. Sarah mentioned to me that the WSIB had approved the use of the Checker taxi for my transportation between my home and the Parkwood. I told Sarah to cancel my daily dinner. After getting the updated from Sarah, my husband left for his work. Soon after that I also left for my home.

After almost five weeks, I woke up in my own home. That was an assuring and relaxing feeling. On the instructions of the hospital, I was staying on the ground floor at the home. Obviously, the medical team wanted me to take precaution whenever I needed to use stairs. Since a washroom was situated on the first floor too, I did not need to use my bedroom, which was on the upper floor. After getting prepared, I called the Checker taxi and went to the Parkwood, where the nurse gave me the medication. Afterwards, I attended the physio lesson and went for a walk with the physiotherapist assistant, Sarah. After the physio class, I put my amplifier for the charging. Meanwhile, I worked on the reasoning and functional math worksheets which were given to me as the homework. I was comfortably sitting in my favourite section, the big lounge. However, I was feeling like I was getting the elementary school graduation practice, because I had to complete all the given tasks within the given deadlines.

As per the medical instructions, I was not using cell phone or telephone, even when I was in the hospital. On my request, the reception called the taxi. It was a pleasant feeling to see the taxi moving towards my home, leaving the hospital. I got settled in the first room and had my dinner, because my husband had his work shift till the evening. I spent my evening quietly sitting in the living room watching the activities in the surroundings. Soon, it was the sleeping time for me, so I went to the bed and closed my eyes effortlessly.

It was an unbelievable fact that in the present age of the modern technology, when people are addicted to cell phones, the Internet, and televisions, I had spent the period of more than five weeks without using any of these devices for. Obviously, it was my deep-rooted desire to get completely recovered that was pushing me for such rough and tough struggle. Otherwise, prior to the accident, these devices had an integral role in my personal and professional lives. I would text and talk to my friends and family. I would do a lot of research on the Internet. Also, I would watch lots of movies and shows on the television.

Now, all those sources of maintaining the social contacts, collecting the information, and enjoying the entertainment were removed from my life. However, I was so delighted for getting back on the track of almost a normal life that I did not have much grudge against those limitations. Rather, I started focusing on other possible creative activities, like making the artistic objects from the recyclable material.

Next day, I worked on a financial activity sheet given to me by my occupational therapist. There were some errors in my submitted work, so the occupational therapist told me to take more time and double check my work. Then, under the supervision of the physiotherapist, I used the exercise bicycle for twenty minutes. Subsequently, the speech therapist gave me the cognitive exercises for the homework. After finishing my all lessons, I asked the nurse for additional medication for the weekend.

Finally, I called the taxi that carried me to the home. After having a short nap, I did some light exercises, following the rules mentioned by the therapists. Nevertheless, doing the physical exercises or completing the homework at the home, in the free atmosphere, where no one was watching around, was a far greater joy. In the hospital, it had strictly the feeling of a student, who was completing the assignments under the supervision of the teachers.

Next day, I was happy that my son came back from Waterloo and was staying with us during the weekend. I knew that he could manage his student life in Waterloo. However, I would take the special pleasure in preparing food for him so that he should not require to cook everyday in the Waterloo cramped kitchen.

When I woke up, my son was still sleeping. I was dusting the furniture when he woke up. After some time, he joined me, and we played few card games. Surprisingly, I won all hands, though I was finding it difficult to focus on the games. While playing the cards, for me the key would be, of course apart from the cheating, to remember the cards that other players would pick up. Certainly, I had not improved much in that area but still I managed to win, especially against my son. Afterwards, we chatted for a while sitting near the Wonderland window, watching the traffic and the pedestrians. Later, we went for the evening walk in our neighborhood and felt relaxed. There were a lot of children around with their heart-warming activities. It would be a fun watching them playing. I observed that my neighbourhood had not changed much in the period of the six weeks when I was in the hospital.

When I woke up, I did some physical exercises prescribed by my physiotherapists and then worked on the homework sheets. My husband joined me in checking the homework. He said that my answers to most questions were correct, though he made some suggestions. I started modifying my answers accordingly. I put back all worksheets into the folder and started arranging the cushions on the sofa. The next day, my son was leaving for Waterloo, so my husband was cooking for him. He was singing a Hindi song and I was wondering at his natural gift. He left for the work after finishing the cooking and cleaning the kitchen. My son was still sleeping in the basement. He had been studying late in the night. The television was still on in the low volume. He has still the habit of studying and sleeping with having the television on in the low volume in the background. That is his childhood habit when he would turn on the cartoon channels but keep playing his toy trains without looking at the television.

Next morning, my husband left for work, after preparing the food for us. My son wanted to leave for Waterloo, after I would start for the hospital. However, I told him to leave early, as later the traffic would get increased. After having the breakfast, I called the Checker taxi that brought me to the hospital. A nurse gave me the medication and asked me about my general well being. Then, the occupational therapist, during the class, asked me about my weekend activities. I explained my all routine and submitted my completed homework. After checking it, she gave me some worksheets to complete. After that I had an appointment with Carley, the speech therapist. After the formal questionings, she told me to prepare a speech on the topic of managing behavioural issues in school. I would get fifteen minutes for the presentation.

Then, there was the physiotherapy class in the small gym. I did the exercise on a bike and felt that I was balancing far better than earlier I would. After finishing all classes and receiving the medication, I called the taxi. As usual, the nurse stayed with me till I departed. At home, I relaxed by taking a brief nap. Then, I had some snacks. In the evening, I walked in front of my house. I was remembering my past walks with my son. I would find the walking always a fun when I had a company. I recalled that after my marriage, I would go for walk with my husband.

Next day, the assistant occupational therapist, Laura, gave me medication setting practice. She had brought a medication box with some small pouches of lentils and grains. I needed to set the pouches as the medicine like a nurse would do for the weekly plan. I did it well as I had seen the nurses performing the same procedure almost everyday. Afterwards, the physiotherapist took me into the big gym. Several patients were doing their different activities. I had to do my exercise on the bike. I did it while keeping the balance. I humorously thought that at least I had started balancing my life to some extend. During the break, the nurse reminded me that I had still that room for use, but I went to the small lounge for having the lunch.

Dr. Alam came and asked about my routine at the home. I provided him with all the information. Then, the speech therapist, Stephanie, asked about my preparation for the presentation that she had assigned to me. I told her few points about the presentation topic. She further asked about my hearing check up appointment. I told her that it was in June. She told me not to return the amplifier till I would get my hearing aid. The nurse gave me the medication before I left. I went to the reception, who called the taxi for me and I came back to the home.

Next day, when I came back to Parkwood, I was informed that my one class had been cancelled. However, as per the schedule, we went to Springbank Park. It was a very beautiful place. We walked around the Springbank Park, using the walkways, which was running parallel to the river. The therapists and assistants asked if I was tired. I said that I was fine. However, I also told them that I would walk a lot in the past, but now I could not. While chatting with them, I kept walking. After the picnic, I went back to my home.

Next day, at Parkwood, I had class scheduled with the occupational therapist. I had to do some math questions and I also had to identify some animal pictures correctly. Next, they told me to draw a clock, showing the indicated timings. I knew that such exercises were essential to fine tune my cognitive skills, but these activities would appear simple to me. After the break, the physio therapist assistant took me for the walking test. In that test, I had to walk fast, keeping my balance intact and come back to the starting point. I was trying to walk as fast as possible in the big lounge. Then, in the next test, I had to close my eyes and cross the corridor, keeping the head in the left position and then keeping it in the right position. The exercise required to go and come back while changing the head positions alternatively. I did the activity moderately well, but I felt I could do it better. During the lunch, to boost my confidence about my body balance, I handled the tray by myself. I went in the other small lounge for the break and did my homework.

After lunch, I had to present on topic of managing behavioural issues at school for 15 minutes. Connie Ferri, the speech language pathologist asked some questions about my topic. I responded in brief keeping my statements attached to the topic. Karley Charrette, the communication disorder assistant, and the student assistant were also present on the scene and were asking some short questions. I was not nervous, but I felt that I was facing an interview at a school board office. Finally, they told me that my presentation was good. Hence, my classes were over for the day. I took my medication and came back to the home by the taxi. Since I was tired for talking too much at the presentation, I rested on my sofa.

Next day, again I had class with physiotherapist. After that, I came to the lounge for doing my homework. While doing it, I saw a toddler sleeping in the lap of his mother. I recalled that my son was only ten days young, when we brought him from the hospital to our home. We put him in the bedroom. The window was open, thus the sun light was entering into the room. He was moving his tiny delicate hands and legs and was making some lovely grunting noises. After some time when his position was changed, the sun light started disturbing him. He could not move and change his position by himself. Thus, he was getting bothered by the sun light, but he was still smiling. We helped him and changed his position to make him more comfortable. I thought that in our childhood we receive the parental care and support in all sorts of problems. However, in our adulthood, we have to take care of ourselves. After lunch, Sarah, the social worker, asked about my wellness and told me that I would get discharged on May 31, and then I would not need to be in hospital every day, though some check ups would be still there.

Next morning, my son had arrived from Waterloo before I woke up. I had the medication before completing the physiotherapist recommended exercises. Then, I joined my family for the breakfast. After a long time, we all three were leisurely dining together, though my husband was about to go for the work, and my son needed to do the studies as his exam was not far away. The rest of the day went in doing the homework and going for the walk with my son in the Chapman area. I enjoyed rest of my weekend as I got to spend lot of time with my family.

Next week was the last one that I had to come to Parkwood for my therapy. So, I was excited to get the week started. My first class was with Melisa, who observed my yoga. Melisa made some notes on my demonstration, and then told me to continue it after my discharge. However, she cautioned me against the acts of running, jumping, or rushing while doing any activity. She told me to avoid time pressure completely and perform all Yoga exercises easily and leisurely. She mentioned to me that there were cognitive limitations with me, and any sudden movement or unexpected jerk could worsen my brain injury.

Soon, it was time for the occupational therapy class. The assistant Laura gave me a worksheet. I tried to focus on it as two other patients were working too in that room. Later, I went to the speech therapy class. Stephanie told me to keep doing the passage reading and question answering exercise after the discharge and gave me some additional worksheets. After finishing my classes, I came back to my home. After reaching home, I called Sameena, Dr Alam's wife and my close friend. She suggested to buy the chocolates for the hospital staff. Then, I called Fatima, another friend, and told her to help me in buying the chocolates. She readily got agreed and picked me from the home in her vehicle. We went together to the Costco, which was close to her house. It was a crowded place and I was feeling uneasy. However, I did not mention it to Fatima. After checking several chocolate types, we bought a chocolate box. I got extremely tired after all that actions, so slept early after I dinned.

When I arrived at Parkwood the next day, I was informed that I would be getting discharge on May 30 instead of 31st, the original proposed date. I was very happy with this good news. Afterwards, during his visit, Dr. Alam recommended me to intake Vitamin D supplement for life as it would provide for bone support. He clarified that it was not for resolving a medical issue, but it was a supplement provision. He generously mentioned that I could call him at his home phone if any problem appeared. He assured me that everything was positive with me for having no vomiting and headache. He also confirmed that I would get the discharge on May 30 because all reports and therapy class performances were satisfactory.

Happily, I went to the speech therapist class, in which Coney gave me some assignments to work on. I completed all worksheets in the given time. After examining my work, she said that my performance was encouraging. However, she also mentioned that I was not fit enough to go to work as a professional. She further added that I would get additional teacher support at home, even after my discharge, so that I should get prepared as a professional. I nodded my head in the acceptance, as there was no other choice. Finally, I gave her the grade eight papers for her son that she asked for some days before.

After the class, I sat near the fountain. Susie, the therapist, approached me and told that she would be at my home for the further classes after I got discharged. She gave her professional card to me. I thanked her. She appeared a nice lady and a competent professional to me. Thus, I was comfortable for having her as the therapist at the home. I came back home soon after that.

I was informed earlier by the hospital that I should be accompanied by a family member on the day of the discharge so that my report could be discussed. However, the hospital later changed the instruction, stating that I could come alone if I was not anxious of reading the self medical report and the assessment of my performance in the therapy classes.

Taking such responsibilities at crucial occasions was not an unfamiliar task for me. I recalled that I had signed the Caesarian form and went to the operation theatre at the juncture of the delivery of my son. In fact, I was with my husband at the hospital for the check up at the last stage of my pregnancy. The doctor told him to bring some test reports from two other hospitals. He left immediately, as the delivery was due at anytime. However, after his departure, the chief doctor of the hospital, in the consultation with other doctors, concluded that I needed the caesarian operation for the delivery. She asked me if I wanted to wait for my husband to return and sign the consent from, though she added that sooner they could start, the better it would be for me and my baby. I made the instant decision, signed myself the form, and went in the operation theatre. By the time, my husband returned with the reports, I delivered my baby. Therefore, reading my injury report could not be a problem for me, despite of having some cognitive damages.

On the day of my discharge, I went to the hospital by Checker taxi. In the physio class, I gave a "Thank You" card to Melissa. She thanked me for my gesture. I completed some gym exercises on her instructions. After watching my physical movements during the exercise, she said that I was doing well, and perhaps I would not need a regular physio therapist support after my discharge. However, she added that the observing team would make the decision in that respect. The occupational therapist gave me an iPad for the last lesson. After the lesson, she said that I was a disciplined patient and followed all the given instructions properly. She told me to take care as I would be on my own most of the time after that day. I could notice the tone of concern, empathy, and affection in her voice. I was also going to miss her. Afterwards, I had an appointment at the Western for the OMFS / Oral maxillofacial services. The assistant helped me in visiting there. On the way, I pleasantly told her with the child like enthusiasm about my discharge. She congratulated me for that but also cautioned to be careful while dealing with the physical movements.

At the Western hospital, which was now quite familiar hence comfortable for me, the doctor checked me after asking some medical background questions. Having examined my all reports, he declared that he found no health issues in the reports. However, the doctor told me to take extreme care, to walk slowly and cautiously, to eat only soft food leisurely, and to avoid all strenuous activities and energetic games. After picking the report from the hospital, I talked to the assistant, who told me to take the same taxi to go to the home via the Parkwood. At Parkwood, I thanked everyone. At that moment, I had the sense of mixed emotions – thoughtful for leaving such compassionate professionals, and ecstatic for getting the liberty of living without much restrictions. Overcoming my surge of emotions, I came back to the home by the same taxi. After arriving at home, I felt I had graduated and was now going to have the much-awaited holidays.

CHAPTER 3

THE RISING PROCESS AT HOME SWEET HOME

The home makes us strong and then we leave it to chase our dreams, but it is only the home where we want to go back when we become weak.

Thursday, May 31, 2018

My Home, Chapman Court, London

AFTER HAVING MY breakfast and medication, I started reading my medical report sitting near the window. I decided to put my body into the action. Thus, I dusted the furniture, then had the lunch, and later a brief nap. After waking up, I found that it was raining so I couldn't go out for walk. So, to keep myself engaged, I took out our family album. I found my son's early childhood pictures along with many other family photographs. He was then only two months old. I was on the maternity leave and would not go to the school for work. One day, I was reading a book, while he was playing nearby. All of the sudden, I noticed that he had closed his eyes, lying on the bed. I tried to get his attention by calling him, and then shaking him, but he did not respond. My husband was at his work, and no one else was at the home. Thus, I decided to take him to the hospital, sensing some health issue. Our house was located nearby a clinic. I took him in my arms and came out. There were some teachers also living around. One of them was Sandhya, who was working as the supervisor in the same school and she was my friend. She was a quiet and kind-hearted lady. When she saw me holding my son in my arms, she inquired about the situation. I told her that my son was not responding and there were no movements in him, so I was taking him to the hospital. Being an experienced mother, she was familiar with such situation. She pushed his body a little harder and he opened his eyes. Still, we went to the doctor, who checked him throughout and declared that he was fine. He added that he might have slept suddenly. Still, as being a mother, I was worried, so the rest of evening, I kept sitting nearby him.

The rain stopped in the late afternoon. Almost all neighbours were at the work, thus, the entire parking lot was vacant. I decided to go for a walk. The sidewalk was most of the time deserted. After few minutes walk, I noticed three elementary kids selling cookies to raise the fund for some noble cause. One of them approached me. I softly told him that I needed to bring my purse in order to contribute. I turned back towards the home and in my next lap of the walk, I gave him some toonies. I was content to see the jubilant smiles of all kids.

June 2018

Once I was back at the home and got settled into my daily routine, the life started moving slowly yet steadily. My only aim was to get recovered from the cognitive damage in order to get back into the workforce. However, nothing could be done immediately about that issue. I thought maintaining an optimistic approach was the key, especially when challenges, like physical or mental weakness, would surface.

During the month, I kept doing the same practices recommended by the physiotherapist, the speech therapist, and the occupational therapist. The weather was turning warmer, rather hotter. The plants started bearing colourful flowers and the leaves were turning bigger, greener, and denser. The birds started chirping louder, and I could see the animals, like bunnies, beavers, squirrels, and racoons in action around, occasionally producing some wonderful sounds. I could watch the kids playing around my home in the colourful dresses, making lovely giggles.

I tried to sleep while recalling my working days in India. I would correct the students' work in the late-night hours, listening the Hindi movies songs. All musical pieces were melodious, but the moments connected to them would make them memorable. Those were my initial teaching days of my first job. I had no other matter of more interest thus I would enjoy the late-night working too. Shabana, my niece, would be the only available but close companion. I smiled at the contradiction. In those days, I would correct the mistakes, but now I was myself making the mistakes. I fell in the hold of the deep sleep while wondering at my reversed role.

On June 14, a day after his birthday, my son was back from Waterloo. He had submitted his all assignments and now was preparing for the exams. I was glad that he did well on his assignments. However, I was disappointed that I could not be with him on his birthday. We would always celebrate his birthday at home. I recalled my sons' first birthday. We had prepared his favourite dishes, including sweets. Then, we also took him to my mom's home. She blessed him affectionately, showering several kisses. She had an exceptional liking for him, perhaps because she would find his face identical to mine.

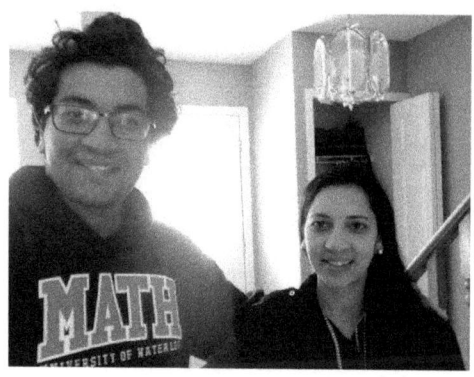

My son after coming back from Waterloo

Afterwards, we took him to my school's principal, who was a professional but kind-hearted lady. My son had a distinct place in her heart. She used to watch his lovely childish activities. Thus, when she saw him on his first birthday, she patted him with affection and gave him some money as the token of blessings. We took a picture of them together. Later, we took him to the gynecologist, who had supervised his delivery. My son was happy after wearing new clothes and having his favourite sweets.

Suddenly, I had a surge of pain inside my heart when I fathomed the wide gulf between my physical ability on his first birthday and my disability on his twenty second birthday. Then, I would move around rapidly, holding him proudly in my arms. However, now I could not even be with him when he was even less than hundred kilometres away from me. Nevertheless, I collected myself thinking that I needed to avoid the surge of such negative emotions if I wanted to cross that wide gulf of disability.

Having familiar with my disability, my son went to the hospital with me on June 15 for the appointment with Dr Parnes at the Western Hospital. I had a light long chat with him that day, as we waited a lot in the waiting room, enjoying the beautiful view of the Western faculties. The attendant called us on our turn. We both went inside. The student doctor asked the usual health related questions. The doctor read my case notes and asked a question, but I had hearing problems so I could not respond properly. Then doctor said that I might need the hearing aids. The doctor had checked me before in the connection with my hearing problems, so he told me to take an appointment with the Western audiologist, Dr Sherry. I got it for July 13, on my coming birthday.

While performing my physical exercise, I recalled that I used to play badminton with my son at the Western gym. It is a very big gym with lot of facilities. While I used to play with my son, I had lot of stamina and I would always try to win games. Sometimes, we would join other players. While playing badminton, I would also have to look up to hit the birdies. However, now after injury I can not move my head too much in that way.

The rest of the month went in doing all the exercises given by the therapists. My husband would invariably stay with me during the night hours. However, he would be mostly at work during the day hours. Gradually, my life was getting settled with the given circumstances, though the therapists were scheduled to take control of my daily schedule from the next month.

July 2018

My son was still in Waterloo for his exams, scheduled in July. Given his busy schedule, it was not possible for him to keep visiting me. My husband was busy with his work during the day hours. I would keep doing all exercises, including the physio ones, that were suggested by the therapists. My therapy classes at home were scheduled to begin from July 4.

The whole plan of the therapy classes was called the Outpatient Therapy. It was made up of Occupational therapy, rehabilitation therapy, and speech therapy. Besides, I needed to follow the instructions given by the physiotherapist and keep doing the recommended physical exercises. The decision-making team had observed that I was precisely following the instructions given by the physiotherapist, hence the regular physio classes were not included into the Outpatient Therapy plan. However, all three therapists – the occupational, the rehabilitation, and the speech – would keep observing my physical movements. They would also suggest any changes based on my strengths and weaknesses.

The schedule for the therapists' visits or classes was roughly divided into three sections. During the first three days of the week, each therapist would visit one day for ninety minutes. I would be visited by the occupational therapist, speech therapist, and rehabilitation therapist on Monday, Tuesday, and Wednesday respectively. However, the plan was flexible, and they could change their visiting days by scheduling themselves for any other weekday. Still, I would get two weekdays free, mostly Friday and some other weekday. The flexibility was designed for the rehabilitation therapy, as the therapist would require planning for outdoor activities. Mostly these activities would also require good weather.

Despite of such well-organised plans and the flexibility, I would often get tired during those classes. However, the therapists would expect such tiredness on my part, as they were well-aware about my traumatic brain injury. Thus, they would go at a slow pace and would allow me some time to relax. Nevertheless, they all told me that they would prepare me for going back to the work and would help me in overcoming the setbacks of the traumatic brain injury. They all were also trying to assist me in coping with the hearing loss by applying their expertise and utilising the hearing aids that I received later.

The first to visit at my home was the occupational therapist, Susan. In fact, she was also present in the final meeting at Parkwood. However, I was so occupied with several other thoughts that I did not notice this kind-hearted therapist then. During her first visit, she mentioned about the speech therapist, Suzie and the rehabilitation therapist, Lani Saarkoppel. I showed Susan my WSIB papers. After reading them carefully, she mentioned that the WSIB was asking for some formal records. Later, she helped me in reading the WSIB notes and arranging papers accordingly. She also informed me that from the next week, Suzie who was the speech therapist, would start visiting weekly.

Susan asked me about my favourite subject, which was organic chemistry. She gave me the hint that she was completely blank in the organic chemistry subject. Perhaps to make me comfortable by providing the sense of authority, she told me to teach her the organic chemistry topics. Knowing that I was away from the teaching practice from long time, she asked if I needed the help in preparing the lesson plan. I thanked her but added that the help might not be needed. I clarified that I would teach her from the beginning, since she had mentioned that she did not know anything about the subject.

The speech therapist, Suzie, came the next day. After the formal introduction, she asked me for my current teaching subject in the schools. Although, as an occasional teacher, I was teaching multiple subjects, I told her that it was math. She stated that in the coming therapy classes, I had to deliver the linear equation lessons to her. She recommended to watch TED videos for improving my focus on the subject and concentration on the teaching method. She gave me some tips and guiding lines on improving as a teacher in the therapy classes, but she also added that watching TED videos was my homework.

The next was the rehabilitation therapist, Lani, to visit. She told me that her immediate task was to make me comfortable in the open-air activities but that did not mean that we would visit the picnic spots. She clarified that we had to choose the places that we needed to visit often in our routine lives, and in which we required to follow certain formalities and rules. Thus, for the outdoor visits, she gave me several options, such as malls and libraries. She informed me that she would observe my walking efficiency, balance of the body, and communication skills, while I would visit these places.

Lani mentioned that these visits were carefully designed, so that I should not feel lonely. Therefore, they were not strictly educational assignments. While spending more time with her, I found out that she was a cheerful and friendly lady. However, she was a committed and thoughtful professional too, as later I realised, when she would not skip her classes even after her hand got fractured.

All three therapists were considerate and competent instructors. They reminded me of those days when I would teach the kids taking the care of all aspects, like selecting the suitable teaching methods for them and suggesting the feedback and corrective measures. However, now I was getting tutored and receiving the feedback and homework that I would do in the afternoons when the therapists would depart.

During the classes, I would often get tired and lose my focus only in the period of twenty minutes, while explaining my favourite topics, like linear equations, to one therapist. Such deterioration in teaching capability was not only a personal loss, but also a professional degradation. I discussed this issue with all therapists, who all told me that the decline in the teaching skill was the direct effect of the brain injury. They also clarified that any quick fix was not applicable in the case of brain injury, but regaining self-confidence was the key. After going though several discussions with the therapists, in which they also asked about my hobbies and mentioned some recommendations, I started managing the small garden in front of the apartment. I also started working on art craft.

I recalled that in India, I would go with Shamim, my elder sister, for purchasing craft material. We would stroll in several shops looking for appropriate material. Then, at home, I would sit hours to make the craft. However, now I could be able to sit only for half hour or so, thus could not remain as active and agile as I used to be in the past.

My birthday was on July 13, but given the current circumstances, the celebration could not be the same as it would be in the old days, especially in India. We would celebrate my birthday at home by preparing goat biryani, which was my favourite dish at that time. My husband would do most of the arrangement, and then we would visit some nearby picnic spot, spending entire day there. It would be a happy family time.

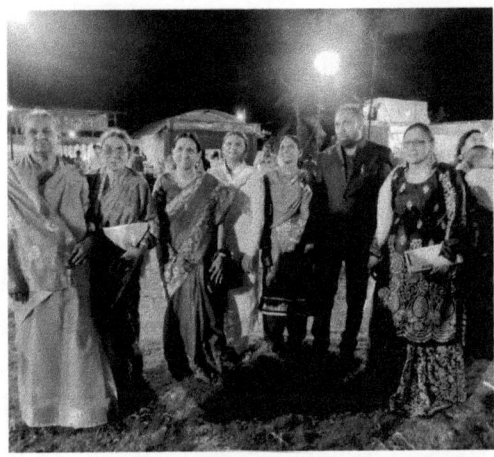

My Family

Anyway, on this birthday, with my son, as per the appointment, after the lunch, I went to visit the audiologist, Sherry, at the Western. She did all medical checks. Then, she showed me the hearing aid sample. She measured my ear size by putting a medical clay piece into my ear. After that she made some notes, and asked me for the type of the aid, in terms of colour and size. I said that I would prefer the black pieces as my hair were black. I also added that I required the small size that could be hidden behind my ears. She noted my preferences and told me that I would get the hearing aids in August. She assured me that she would call me upon receiving the delivery of the hearing aids. I had the hearing problem, so a clear conversation was difficult with her.

However, she needed to collect more information, so she talked to my son as he had most of the information about my medical history.

I informed all my therapists that I would get hearing aids sometime in August. On July 23, the rehabilitation therapist Lani took me to Parkwood Main building, Unit B. The speech therapist was also there. A nurse asked for the details about the therapy classes, the hearing aid, and my progression with the therapists at home. I provided her with all account of the past three months.

Then, Dr Keith Sequeira came to check me. He was a humble, caring and skillful professional, who made me feel comfortable. The speech therapist was still there to support me, if required. The doctor asked for the symptoms that would appear while working longer with the therapists. I could not mention exactly all symptoms but told him that I would get tired quickly. He mentioned that it was because of the brain injury and took my several tests – walking, figure making, etc. My clock making test went wrong as I could not hear him properly. He also found me badly tired, so he gave me a form, and told me to go empty stomach for the blood test. He said that he would contact me if he found something wrong or even worthy to discuss in my blood test report. He asked about my driving skill. I told him that I was prohibited for driving. He sympathetically shook his head and advised to follow the instructions of the therapists. Finally, he gave me the next appointment after one month.

I was under pressure after getting instructions for so many tests, and a big "WHY" started hovering on my head, generating several doubts. However, having received the instructions from the doctor, I went for the blood test with my son. Nevertheless, the lab did not call me even after a week, so I concluded that all was well at least with the blood test.

The rest of the month went eventless, except, our neighbours, who had two lovely kids moved to another house, as they needed a bigger house for their growing kids. I kept attending the therapists' lessons, doing homework and walking during the evening hours on the Chapman sidewalks. My son and husband would accompany me in their free time. The warm weather was certainly motivational in keeping me in the positive state of mind.

August 2018

One of the regular yet significant event of the month was my husband's birthday, though we formally never celebrated it. In the early years of our marriage, I was keen to prepare some dishes and arrange a gift for him, but after finding him indifferent about his birthday gifts, I modified my approach towards his birthday celebration. We would visit nearby picnic spots on his birthdays, if we had off time from the work. Nevertheless, he would buy the gifts for me on my birthdays, after asking my preferences.

All the therapists would keep telling me that a brain injury could have a greater impact, sometimes less physical and more psychological, on the patient. However, in my case, they all agreed that the brain injury had negatively affected me in both ways. They, like my doctors, would also mention that the psychological impact might appear in the form of the late chain reaction - no outstanding instant effect, but it starts appearing after a few days, one negative impact leading to another.

I was glad that I had the support of three therapists, each on one weekday. Sometimes, I would feel like I was going through a tiresome routine but overall it was a beneficial provision. At least, my there days were occupied by the therapists in order to get rid of those needless worries. Still, I had two weekdays and the weekends free, but I would utilize them for doing additional physical exercises, though I would do the physio exercises everyday.

It was still the summer like weather, the trees were filled with green leaves and colourful flowers. The wind was still warm, though occasionally, especially during the rain, it would turn a little colder. I would think that in India, August would bring a lot of rain. Students would go to school wearing the colourful raincoats. They would get the rain days, as here, in Canada, the students get the snow days. In India, my son would have to stay at home in a heavy rain day, and I would teach him giving him several exercises to practice as the homework. I was a loving mother, but I would also play the role of a strict teacher, indeed for the betterment of his future. However, he was an obedient student, thus I never needed to force him for his studies.

I inherited such strict approach because my parents and elder sister were firm about my studies. The education was not only the medium of securing a promising career for our middle-class family, but also a way of living an organised life. Thus, inheriting those qualities from my family, I was quite thoughtful about my son's education. However, I never compared him to his classmates nor pushed him to be number one. My goal was to keep improving him everyday as a student. In fact, his school admission was in itself a wonderful experience.

He was still away from his fourth birthday, when he got admitted in the school. I was worrying about his school interview, as he would barely speak a few clear sentences. However, the process went smoothly, because the principal knew my husband, who used to visit the school because of the professional reasons. Thus, my son was not asked any question during the interview.

Nevertheless, in the company of other students, my son started speaking quickly, and turned into a chatter box. I took the task of monitoring his studies as a self-imposed mission. Even I would sacrifice my evening walks for some days to be with him. For the sake of his studies, I would not mind leaving my professional and social activities and staying at home. Now, I was strict on myself for following the instructions delivered in the therapy classes because doing studies meticulously for the success was a well trodden path for me.

Nonetheless, my motherly instinct was still intact despite of being a patient of the brain injury and a student under the scanner of the therapists. I was still a mother, who was the source of inspiration and support for my son. Accepted that after having the traumatic brain injury, I was not as energetic as I used to be, still he would approach me in his moments of uncertainty.

My son was going to start his job on August 20. We all were happy and celebrated at home. Then, I went a store with my husband and bought several items, like a water bottle, a bag, a lunchbox and so on, for him so that he could go to the office prepared. I had bought almost the same items for him when he was going to the school on the first day. For me, his first day at the school and the first day at the job were equally significant.

The next day, on August 21, as it was informed by the office of the audiologist, I got the hearing aids at the Western hospital at 5 pm. With my son, I went to Sherry, the audiologist, who said that after the injury, my both ears were partially functioning - the fourteen percent of the right ear and the seventy six percent of the left ear. She demonstrated the hearing aids showing how to use them. My son also practiced with the doctor.

Sherry told me to use those hearing aids gradually, increasing their application. She alerted me that I would initially feel headache for not having practice of using the hearing aids. She also told me to be back to her clinic for getting my ears rechecked. Since I had the hearing problem, I could not follow all her instructions clearly. Therefore, my son explained all instructions to me.

We came back to the home from the Western and did some more practice with the hearing aids. Later, I told the therapist about receiving the hearing aids and requested her to return the amplifier to the Parkwood. However, at the same time, I had the negative thoughts that how I would accommodate with the hearing aids by adjusting the setting as per the requirement. Such uncertainty emerges when someone deals with a new equipment or machine, especially when it is going to be a supporting part of one's essential senses. I had also the thought that using the hearing aids was a sort of permanent handicap. It was a harsh reality, a permanent sense damage. Thus, like any normal person, I was reasonably anxious.

During the month, the doctors would call me for the monthly check up and I would keep going by the taxi that would bring me back too. The occupational therapist would go with me as she needed to collect the report. The school board would keep inquiring about my status, and the board receptionist would keep inspiring and assuring me that the things would be fine. I was grateful for her kind words, but now I had more realistic approach.

September 2018

It was the official beginning of the fall season. However, the weather was still comfortably warm. Trees started shedding few yellow leaves. The biggest change was the flowing wind, which would sometimes transform into a temporary minor storm. Mostly, the sky would be clear, though the occasional rain would make the earth wet. I would not get disturbed by such slight changes in the Nature as that would least affect my outdoor activities. However, the activity I would miss badly was going to work. I had been a teacher since my early twenties. Back in India, I would tutor the students before joining the school as a teacher. After getting teacher's certificate, I started working as a teacher till I immigrated to Canada. Thus, teaching job was an addiction for me. Like other professionals, I would like to go on vacations. Nevertheless, I would have a keen desire to resume the teaching work on the arrival of July, the opening month for schools in India.

After arriving in Canada, my schedule got changed as the first week of September was the starting point for the teaching job. Therefore, by the end of August, I would keep prepared my clothing and vehicle. Those preparation processes were the inevitable parts of my routine, like eating and sleeping. As they say, a journey is more enjoyable than the point of arriving at the destination. However, in that respect, I had lost both, the journey as well as the destination. Thus, I was not melodramatic in missing my preparation to go to work.

Although it was an internal battle that I needed to win it on my own, the therapists would provide me the external support. However, as it is said, all good and bad matters come to an end. The speech therapist, Suzie informed me that she got a job elsewhere. She also told me that some other therapist would replace her and would come to teach me shortly. She gave me some additional worksheets to work on till the next therapist would resume her work. She assured me that it would be a smooth transition as she would hand in my progress report with all details and recommendations to the next therapist. However, it was not a comfortable feeling to lose her services as I had established a harmony with that experienced professional.

At that moment, I had two therapists, the rehabilitation and the occupational, visiting weekly. I would get several worksheets from both that would keep me busy. I would recall my teaching practices when I would give my students several homework sheets. Suzanne, the occupational therapist, would keep bringing new ideas of learning for me, apart from implementing her customary instruction procedures. Since she was the in-charge of the entire Outpatient Therapy plan, she would monitor my progress in other classes too. In her process of assessing my abilities to rejoin the workforce, she would deliver her lessons steadily and would give me consistent homework. However, she would not force me to speed up. As per her instructions, I would teach her the organic chemistry subject for the brief period in each occupational class, but I was not satisfied with my performance even after teaching her in the several periods.

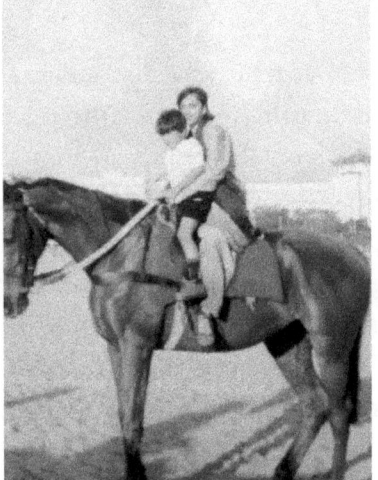

Riding Horse
without afraid of falling

Nevertheless, the practice of regular physio exercises started showing the positive impact as my physical strength and the level of body balance were improving. Subsequently, I would do light indoor work, like cooking and cleaning, independently, but I was still not permitted for driving, performing the job work, and going for outing alone.

To give me the required professional behavioural experience, Lani, the rehabilitation therapist, would take me to the various malls and libraries. While riding in her vehicle, I observed that she was a safe driver. However, she told me that some of her clients got paranoid after their accidents and were scared to board with her in her vehicle. During my visits to the malls and the libraries, she would demonstrate how to perform formally certain tasks. She would encourage me to communicate with others. To cope with my hearing loss, I would take my hearing aids everywhere.

On her instructions, I would assist her in dealing with her clients and patients. Among her clients, there was a girl, who was not doing well in maths, so I demonstrated her how to solve the fraction problems by drawing circles and folding papers. Observing my teaching methods, Lani expressed that I was quite good in maths. Taking the advantage of her encouraging words, I told her that for the homework, I would do more maths related problems, but the word puzzles were not exciting for me. She patted my hand after hearing that. She knew that I was still far away form gaining the lost professional efficiency, though she would never mention it to me. Meanwhile, the school board would keep asking about my status and progress, but the board officials would also know that I was far below than the expected level to resume the job duties.

I would have regular doctor appointments. During my medical check ups, the doctor cautioned me that my weight should not go above fifty-five kilogram because gaining the excess of weight could cause additional health problems. However, he also added that my weight should not go very low, because a slender physique would not provide me the much-needed energy. I noticed that I started gaining weight for two reasons. Firstly, I had lost my physical movements because of the accident. Secondly, I would only consume food recommended by the hospital. Indeed, the hospital suggested menu would help in gaining the strength, but it was also high on the calories. Thus, I changed my regular diet by eliminating meat and sweets.

My son was busy with his office work, and his schedule would not permit him to spend much time with me during the weekdays. My husband was engaged in his job duties having long working hours, so he would mostly sleep when he would be at home. However, their busy schedules would not bother me much. I was in my home having the freedom of choosing my activities and not in the hospital, where my activities were restricted, guided and scheduled.

In my free time, I would keep walking on the side walks of my neighbourhood. I would see some kids playing in the small garden. That scenario would remind me my son's childhood activities in the garden when he was barely two-year old. He would be reluctant to slide, and I would assist him in sliding, by holding him on stairs and catching him at the end of the slide. However, now he would support me in the theatres when I would use the stairs. It was the reversal of the roles.

The brain injury and the hearing loss would keep hovering over my cognitive loss that permanently stationed against my professional skills. That awareness would make me feel a deep pain inside. My realistic thinking would not allow me to believe that the pain stops bothering you if it stays for long time inside you. However, I had found my ways to ignore that pain by keeping myself engaged in the meaningful activities that would make me realize that my utility was not over yet.

October 2018

The month started with some infrequent movements around. Our one neighbour, who had earlier three university students as the tenants sold out his apartment. The new buyer was a family having three lovely kids. These neighbours would keep telling me to have the rest and to work slowly. I would clarify that staying stay at one place for long would make me uneasy, thus I needed to move around and work. Their younger son would always watch me sitting on the Wonderland chair. I would give him candies, and he would joyfully go back to the home.

Partially influenced by our neighbours, we started contemplating on the idea of moving to a bigger house. My artistic interest and gardening hobbies, which were also my support system in fighting against the brain injury negative impacts, would encourage me to move in a bigger house. Gardening for me was like nurturing the infants and upbringing the toddlers. Watching plants growing and taking their care was the process that would provide me the inner strength in fighting against the negative psychological impact of the brain injury. My therapists would also confirm my feelings and would encourage me to have interest in the gardening.

In addition, several artistic plans were circling in my mind about setting a spacious house. It was like putting my soul into it. On the suggestions of the therapists, I started creating craft arts that would assist me in diverting my attention away from my inactivity. This psychological healing process was showing its positive effect on my mentality as I would often find myself in a pleasant composure. Besides, since childhood, I had to live in a moderate housing, where I would share all spaces with my siblings. Thus, I did not want to miss the opportunity of having a spacious house of my own.

The new speech therapist, Adrienne, started visiting weekly replacing Susie. Despite of receiving my report card and the subject history with Susie's recommendation, she started her lessons from the basics. After discussing with me about my interest, she declared that there would not be any puzzle solving exercises. She accepted that the given clues could be difficult for me to analyze. I was glad that she planned her lessons considering my interests. The other two therapists continued their lessons with the same plans. They both maintained that I was improving gradually.

Apart from the therapists, I had one more regular visitor – our property agent, David Aspinall. He was a cheerful, talkative, and active person. He helped us in buying our existing house. He would keep providing us with many useful pieces on information even after finishing the purchasing process of the current house. Overall, he was an honest professional with serious approach towards his job. He told us several nitty-gritties related to buying a new house and selling the old one. However, my biggest satisfaction was that he could not identify, despite of our long discussions, that I was a patient suffering from the brain injury.

My son, who would support me in moving, and I would go with

the property agent to visit the houses available for selling. We saw some open houses but did not like them for their structures, sizes, and prices. Some houses were appealing but the surrounding was not appropriate. I had several friends nearby our existing house, and I wanted the new house in the nearby area. Talking to them in my free time would make me feel that I was not a patient anymore. The therapists too had encouraged me to have increasing social contacts to fight against the damaging psychological impact of the brain injury. Besides, the nearby area to the existing house would be closer from my son's office. I conveyed my preferences to the property agent, and he assured that he would narrow his search on the houses available in the neighbouring areas.

Meanwhile there was the monthly medical appointment with Dr. Siqueira. The therapist would always come with me for my medical appointments to collect the report and to ensure my safety. The doctor gave me some tips to keep the blood sugar and the cholesterol within the limit. He told me that I was doing fine but also prohibited me from driving and going alone outdoors. He was satisfied that I was following all given medical advises meticulously.

Halloween was fast approaching. To celebrate the festival, I took a picture with my husband in the Halloween hat. On this event, the kids from colony, including my neighbours' both sons, would visit to get the candies. However, on that occasion the youngest son did not show up. I asked his mother and she told me that he had his leg in the plaster. She brought him in her lap. Despite of the broken leg, he was smiling. I gave him the candies which he happily accepted. To keep the memory of the festival, I wanted to take a picture of the large, orange coloured pumpkin but could not do that as my husband and son were busy, and I was not allowed to go outdoor alone. Thus, I needed to suppress my curiosity till the next October.

By the end of the month, on the instructions of the realtor, I started cleaning the Chapman apartment to sell. My son and husband would help me in the cleaning whenever they would be free. When we moved from Platt's Lane, I cleaned the entire apartment on my own. However, my brain injury had made me to seek some help in the cleaning.

I called the professional cleaners to get cleaned the apartment. Also, I told the therapists that the classes might be cancelled as the probable buyers might visit. All three therapists had no issue in cancelling the scheduled classes, but they told me that I needed to inform them in advance. Whenever a buyer visited our house, I would remain sitting in my car in the parking lot and wait as I could not go away alone. I was gladly surprised that our house got sold quickly.

November 2018

The weather started getting colder at the beginning of the month itself. There was the forecast of the snowfall in the middle of the month. Sometimes, we could witness black ice-covered roads in the morning. Although our Chapman apartment got sold, we did not find the new house yet. Our property agent got the grace period for the shifting, though he suggested us not to hurry for buying the new house if we did not like one. Immerse in such thinking, I would keep visiting several houses with my son, and keep discarding them for some or other reasons. It was appearing that buying the new house might not be possible immediately. At that point, the property agent called us to visit an open house.

Coincidentally, my husband and son both were at home. My husband had to go to work after an hour, but he decided to accompany us. As soon as my son saw the house, he liked it. We explored the entire house. My husband told us to have a closer and careful look at the house before making a decision. Along with my son, I liked the house too, though the price was a little high. My husband left but called us after two hours. My son expressed his desire to buy that house. Thus, my husband told us to place the offer. In the next three days, we finalized all formalities as our offer was accepted.

I mentioned our shifting to the new house to all therapists, who gave me fifteen days off period for moving to the new house. They all discussed with each other about my case and chalked the further plan for me. I was glad that they told me that there would be no driving test till the next year. I was not sure about my cognitive capabilities, stamina, and will power, so I thanked them. I also conveyed them my new address, and got it updated in all other records.

For Remembrance Day, in schools we would wear poppy and pay respect to people who have served our country. I was not in school, but I was wearing poppy to respect the people.

On November 14, we visited the lawyer's office who made us sign some papers and explained the terms and conditions. He asked about our professions and upon knowing that I was a science teacher who would teach math too, he concluded that I was the mastermind behind buying of the new house. He congratulated me for my wise choice. He did not know that I was moving around with the support of my family and therapists and was guided by the medical team. It was a great feeling to find honour in the eyes of some high professional. For the moment, I forgot my limitations and inability caused by the brain injury.

On the same day, I had the appointment with Dr Sequeira. I told him about my low energy level that would make me tired quickly. He suggested for some supplements, but I declined the intake of medicines. He suggested the option of diet change that I accepted. However, he cautioned that I would gradually improve, so I should not get disappointed finding no significant improvements quickly. I knew that for the sake of the long-term achievements, I had to bear some short-term losses. Therefore, I did not get discouraged for not having an immediate improvement.

The increasingly turning cold weather had put limitations on my physio exercises. I was unable to go on outdoor walks. Thus, on the guidance of the therapists, I would do only indoor walk. Initially, I did not feel any difficulty, but later I found out that the outdoor walk would bring more variation and enthusiasm. However, it was not possible to challenge the weather.

As it was scheduled, Lani took me to a craft workshop, where elderly people were performing several art related activities, like knitting, designing, drawing, etc. I felt an inner joy watching them in action. However, I told Lani that I could not work on craft related activities for long period and would feel pain in my eyes. She assured me that it was not a medical issue. She added that I would feel uncomfortable because I did not perform an extended minute sitting work from long period and there was a sudden change in my physical movement plan. She further explained that she would change the therapy plan for me by including sitting exercises like Yoga that would improve my posture and focus.

On November 15, in the noon, my husband brought a moving truck from a near by company office. I assisted him in putting things into the truck. Our neighbour came to help us out, but we politely thanked him and declined his offer. At the new house some formalities were still being carried out, so we would be able to collect the keys from the lawyer's office only after 5 pm. My son was going to do that while coming back from his office. When the truck was full and locked, I childishly asked my husband if we could park the truck in the parking of the new house. In fact, I was too exited after finding this new mission at my hand to resist my impatience. He explained that we could not do that as per the rules. He left for his work, and I went to take a nap as I had lost my energy. Nevertheless, my mind was clear, and there was no confusion or fatigue. My son came in the evening and we drove the truck to the new house. He was so energetic in the idea of shifting that he started moving the boxes from the truck rapidly. It started snowing that soon converted into the long-lasting flurries. My husband joined us after his shift, and we moved out the remaining things too. We kept doing shifting till 3 am. Then my son decided to stay in the Chapman apartment as the cleaners were scheduled to clean the apartment in the morning. I ate a slice of pizza at the Chapman, which was my last act there.

My husband returned the moving truck the next morning. My son had taken off from the office, so he was helping me at the new house in arranging the rooms. Since I had no therapy classes, I spent the whole day in decorating the house. It was the endless task, and it is still continuing after the passing the period of more than one year.

By the end of the month, the school board asked for the updates. I provided them with the details that were provided to me by my medical team. I thought that I was unable to join the workforce, but now I had a meaningful mission at my hand – to arrange the new house setting, converting it into a home sweet home. It was providing the much-required significance to my life.

December 2018

We almost settled in the new house, though I was still working on arranging some rooms. The basic changes I fond from the Chapman to the new housing were a few. Firstly, the Wonderland window was replaced by the Oxford window from where I could have a panoramic sight of the city, providing the views of several buildings, a rail track, numerous moving vehicles, and the sunrise. Secondly, the small garden was replaced by two big gardens – the front one, which I decorated with the hard work, and the backyard one, which was mostly covered with the lush green grass. Thirdly, the limited indoor plants setting of the Chapman was replaced by several indoor plants with the variety that I arranged from several garden shops. Fourthly, my Yaris got a permanent parking spot in the indoor garage, thus I did not need to remove the accumulated snow over it.

Anyway, the new house was keeping me engaged as it was quite big and would require my serious attention. The stairs were extremely safe thus I would feel secured. My washroom was well-equipped and spacious so I would feel comfortable while using it. Since my husband had put television near the kitchen too, I would enjoy the music while performing my physio exercises. Like the Chapman surroundings, this area was also filled with several kids. It was a delight to watch their child-like funny activities around the school bus. We had nice families around, so I gifted them some chocolates to welcome the new neighbours.

I started receiving help in arranging my new house. Lani would take me to several shops for searching and buying the decoration material. Naheed and Sameena helped me in finding new ways of interior decoration by providing their valuable tips. The therapists would encourage me to keep myself engaged in the new setting plans. Overall, my all free time was getting consumed in arranging the new residence.

My therapy classes started again. Surprisingly, after the first heavy snowfall, there were only occasional flurries. Still, the weather was turning colder with the passing of each day. Thus, the therapist had replaced my outdoor walk in open by the YMCA indoor walk. Lani would take me there every Friday. It was a beautiful place with many indoor walking ramps. The walkers around would encourage me to put more efforts. Other therapists would also give me regular lessons and practices in their subject area. I was glad that the therapists had canceled my driving practice schedule and subsequently the expected driving test because of multiple light but frequent snowfalls.

My son prepared an extremely nice plan for the Key West tour. We were supposed to leave in the late afternoon of December 21 and would be back sometimes at the late night of December 30. The doctors and the therapists permitted me for the tour, mentioning that such outing was essential for me to improve my confidence level and to get connected with the world. They all were confident that I would be safe with my family while travelling. However, they had given me some extended medication with some useful tips. Overall, they had trust in my disciplined lifestyle.

My son left early morning for his job on December 21, thus I packed the luggage and put it in the vehicle with the help of my husband. We picked up my son from his office in the late afternoon and drove towards Detroit, where we had the early dinner. I praised my husband for choosing the eatery catering such delicious food. Then, we bought some food, including my preferred items. The rest of the night I was sleeping on the back seat of the vehicle whereas my son on the front, and my husband was driving. In the morning, we used the washrooms of the rest area, and I had my medicines after having a light breakfast. The area was surrounded by trees and hills. We took some pictures there. At that moment, I was comfortable with myself thus filled with the enthusiasm. There is no point in traveling if you are not enjoying it.

In the late afternoon, we arrived in downtown of Atlanta. I was walking for such long distance after a long time, thus started feeling tired. Noticing my inconvenience, my husband altered the plan. We went to the hotel. I slept skipping the dinner. However, my husband brought the south Indian food and we all had the dinner together. I went to sleep feeling better.

In the early morning, we went for a morning walk around the nearby area, which was appearing like a hill station, having ups and downs. Nevertheless, the temperature was so low that I felt uncomfortable. We came back to the hotel room. My son was still sleeping. Knowing that I needed an early breakfast to have my medication, my husband joined me at the breakfast table. The rest of the day I did not feel any weakness, though we visited several spots, including the Coca Cola building, which was wonderfully decorated with thousands of balloons, and a magnificent fish aquarium, where some extra-large beautiful fishes were swimming in a gigantic circular glass pond.

The next day, we landed in the Tampa zoo, an exciting place having several animals and playful birds. After getting fresh in the hotel, we went to a park, located on a beach, and near a busy airport, thus every minute a plane would keep flying overhead. We came to an Indian restaurant for the dinner, and then went back to the hotel. The next day we spend in three different aquariums. One of them was located on an island and driving there was a thrilling experience. I allotted full marks to my son for choosing such nice place. Finally, we headed towards Key West.

My husband and son drove through majority of the night, Even before entering Islamorada, the road converted into a long bridge, providing the illusion of the vehicle lading into the ocean. We could see only water on the both sides of the road. The view would give the impression that the road would sink into the water. Since after Islamorada, there was not any big station till Key West, my husband stopped near a café. The breakfast did not suit me. After half an hour, when we were enjoying walking on a long bridge, having sea breeze softly patting us, I started feeling the severe stomach pain. My husband and son were suggesting different solutions, but by the time we arrived at Key West, my pain was gone. The rest of the day we were walking on the beach. I enjoyed a wedding being conducted nearby.

The next day was spent in an amusement park. I enjoyed the train ride, which would pass close to the several animals sections. After having the lunch, I put my head on my son's shoulder and had a brief nap. The next day we consumed on the Miami beach. I did not enter the water but did a lot of walk. At the evening, we went to a pizza hut. The doctors categorically told me not to remain empty stomach. The next destination was the Sea-World. It presented several interesting events, including skiing, dolphin show and so on. Some of the skiing acts were unbelievable, like a girl jumping and keeping the balance only on one foot or a boy spinning himself having a girl on his shoulder. The audience kept clapping. My son enjoyed the rides too, I was not comfortable on rides before my brain injury so riding them now was out of the question for me. However, I admired two specific shows there. First, the sea creatures that would behave like humans, especially splashing the water around to tease the audience. Second, a clown who was wisely fooling around imitating several visitors from different age groups applying his marvellous presence of mind. There was a good lighting show at the evening that would make us believe that we were passing through a cave filled with thousands of stars.

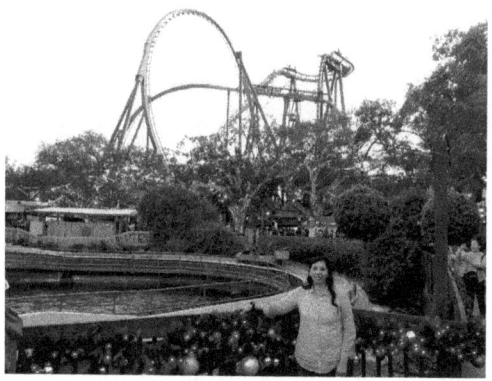

My first vacation after injury

Finally, it was time to head back towards our city. On the way we enjoyed the road passing through the beautiful mountains. While driving through Cincinnati, we had the view of several towering illuminating buildings. There was an exceptionally decorated and inviting casino building too. We crossed Sarnia quickly as there were not many vehicles. I was surprised how fast the time had flown away. We were planning to have the hot home-made food after arriving at the home. However, it was 2 am so we straight went to the beds.

This month was the most pleasant one for me after having the brain injury. True that my health issues were still there, but this outing brought back my self-belief. At one point, after the brain injury, I would think that the real-life fun was over for me, and from here on I had to live only formally, following the medical instructions. I had got the required "push" to move forward with some purpose.

January, 2019

The new year reminded me that I had crossed the tough period of nine months after my accident. I managed to get through with the support of my family and friends, and the guidance of the therapists. With the beginning of the new year, my therapy classes came back to the normal schedule.

The Speech therapist, who was observing my communication skill from a considerably long period and was preparing report on it, came to YMCA walking ramp with the rehabilitation therapist to observe how I manage to communicate with her. After the rehabilitation walking session, she told me that my speaking skill appeared low as I could not reply to others' questions fluently. However, she added that my communication skill was not that low as my hearing ability was. I explained to her that I could not respond immediately as I could not pick up certain words from unfamiliar voices despite having the hearing aids.

She had also mentioned that there was not much improvement in my walking style because I was still extra careful while walking. She added that perhaps I did not possess the required body balance. I clarified that the doctors were satisfied with my body weight, and I would keep doing all physio exercises without feeling any inconvenience. She patted on my hand and assured me that I would achieve my previous walking style if I keep continuing my efforts. Despite of her encouraging words, I thought why I could not notice my defective walking manner in the past one month. However, she was the professional, and she knew better. I told myself if I wanted to improve, I should not defend myself against the professionals' advice. If I kept justifying my act and declining the given feedback, then I would not be able to add the required corrective measures in my performance.

On my health issues, Dr. Alam and Dr Makenzie would come up with some easy and applicable solutions. I recalled that on the day of my discharge from the Parkwood, I could not meet Dr Makenzie, as she was on leave. I met Dr. Alam and presented a plant to him as a token of appreciation. I was grateful for Sameena, Naheed and Fatima's contribution, as they would keep calling and meeting, despite of their busy schedule. Therefore, I met them to express my gratitude. Some of my students and their parents came to meet me, as they could not meet me after my discharge.

I had to arrange several pieces of furniture to set my house. I would go with my son in various furniture shops to order the furniture. After talking to my husband, I arranged a table tennis set at home. It was the best investment as we keep utilizing it till the present day. After long work, it is a great relief to have an indoor physical activity, when we cannot go the outdoors to walk or play in the cold weather. Sameena would also take me for the shopping, though she would be busy as her home was getting renovated. She and Naheed were close friends and always helped me.

February, 2019

The month was filled with occasional incidents of heavy snowfall, though the temperature would remain moderate. My son would keep shoveling the snow from our driveway and would keep reminding me not to come out in the snow. However, to provide my visiting therapists a safe walking passage, sometimes I would clear the doorsteps, which was not risky at all.

Adrienne, had noticed my defective walking style in the previous month. Thus, she recommended for a regular physiotherapist. As a patient, I was required to follow certain formalities, like attending the classes on the scheduled time, completing certain medical check ups, keeping my diet under the control, and most tiring was doing all paper works, including a lot of homework. It would seem like I was back to the elementary school as a student, where life was not easy for me.

I was reluctant about resuming the driving practice and eventually going for the driving test. As per the last Outpatient assessment, I was supposed to resume the driving practice sometime in the last week of the March, depending on the severity of the snowfall, and then I had to go for the driving test in the April. However, after discussing my health status with all three therapists and upon receiving their recommendations, I declined to go for the driving test in the April. I mentioned the genuine reason that I could not remain in the sitting position in a vehicle for the period of one-hour and forty-five minutes that was required for the driving test. I might be confident about my driving skill but not sure about remaining active in the driver's seat for almost two hours and committing no mistake. At that point, I did not possess the required focus and the physical strength. In turn, I was rather prepared to attend all therapy classes, and keep making notes for them.

Visiting the Parkwood would be an inspirational experience because it would remind me of my tough struggling days that I had successfully faced. I visited Parkwood hospital as I had an appointment with Dr. Sequeira. After our my conversation he assured me I was doing good. However, he mentioned that the cardio exercises must be gradually increased. When I asked about my body weight, he assured me that I was doing well in that respect. I recalled Dr Alam's polite and inspiring words that being underweight was not an advantage because the body should support the recovery process of the patient.

March 2019

All the therapists started visiting regularly, with their lessons, homework and feedback. I would mostly complete the physiotherapist recommended exercises at the home, though in good weather I would visit the outdoor ramps with the therapists. There was no change in my health status so far and my doctors too did not recommend any additional check ups.

The month made me recalled that it was the period of the school board exams in India, a significant juncture for a teacher. Since I was an administrator too, I needed to apply my all cognitive skills to manage the board officials, to schedule the invigilators, and to conduct the school office. That was a learning curve, bringing a lot of stress, but that also transfigured me into a mature professional. However, at present, a single event of the brain injury had snatched my all cognitive skills, maturity, experience, and courage, bringing me back to the starting line of the race of my professional life.

The month had one more significant day for me, as 20 March was the death anniversary of my parents. My father passed away in in 1986, and my mother joined him in 2000. They were a perfect couple having some similarities and differences.

My father was an intellectual professional, a chartered accountant, whereas my mother was a modest homemaker. However, they both would value the education quite highly. The father was a strict observer of the happenings around him and would take great pain for my studies. He would help me in going to and coming back from the school and later from the college. He would talk to my friends about their studies in the length so that he could collect the updates on my companions. My mother would make me sit and study on her bed when I was younger to ensure that my studies would remain above the required level. My father was an affectionate person and would lovingly chatting with me despite of his busy schedule. My mother was a loving parent too. In my childhood, she would tell me to climb on the table and would take me into her lap. Both would scrutinize my activities but would also allow me to play with my friends either in our or their home. They would trust us in allowing to go for the outings and the movies.

My parents taught me to remain positive in all situations, as they would maintain that even a bad phase of life would pass sooner or later. Their optimistic approach towards the life helped me in facing the difficulties in the hospital and fight against the adversities brought by the brain injury. They both would inspire me to excel in the studies so that I could achieve a substantial professional position in my life. They both would value their time and would keep engaging themselves in one or other work. After his retirement, he would keep accepting the private accountancy work that would keep him busy. I rarely found him engaging in the time killing activities, like chatting. She had the same policy about the time management. She would also keep helping my elder sister in running her classes.

They both had a strong determination while dealing with the social pressure. We had several relatives around, having traditional lifestyle with conservative attitude. Most of them were averse of providing the high education to the girls. My parents would never pay attention to their comments and would keep protecting us against the social pressure.

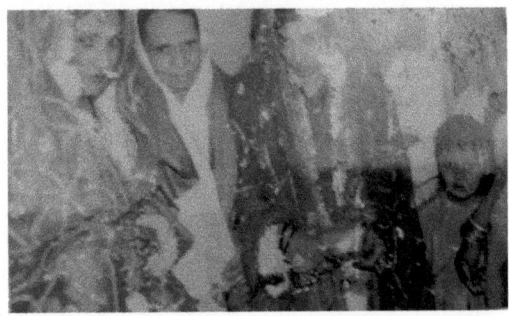

My mother at wedding

Nevertheless, despite of my positive approach, some or other hurdles would keep appearing in the way of recovery from the brain injury. I would keep monitoring my body weight. I found that I got it increased despite of controlling my diet. My body weight was 49 kilograms before the accident, but it was 54 kilograms, while getting discharged from the hospital. The medical recommendations would keep telling me to gain physical strength for fighting against the brain injury issue.

Before having the brain injury, I was obsessed with the objective of keeping my body into the shape. Since, I was free to perform all sorts of exercises, for not having any serious health issue like the brain injury. However, now to keep my body into the shape, I had to control my diet under the guidance of the dietician and perform only the exercises recommended by the medical team.

Meanwhile, Susan, the occupational therapist was replaced by Heather, as the former went on her maternity leave. Despite of this replacement, all therapists were working in the coordination and were looking for a family doctor for me. Lani tried with most of the medical groups though I could not get family doctor. My therapist found Lisa, a dietitian for me. Adrienne was with me when I went for the appointment with the dietitian.

After checking my previous blood report, the dietitian said that she would seek my fresh blood report. However, she made some suggestions for making changes in my diet and keeping cholesterol under the required level. When I told her that I would get tired soon, she explained that my previous blood report was normal, so the tiredness could be the result of some sort of excessive work.

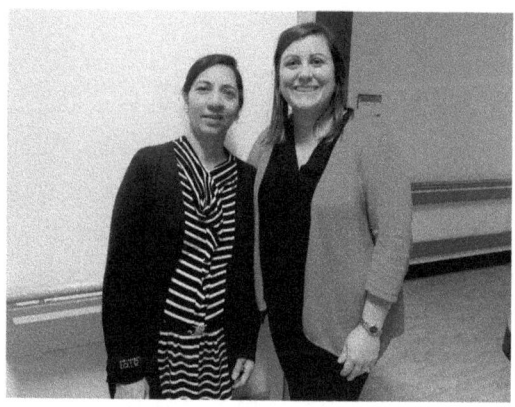

My outpatient speech therapist, Adrienne

Her comments about the excessive work were taken seriously by my therapists' team. They had a comprehensive discussion about the workload that I would get to complete during the therapy classes and after that as the homework. Finally, they decided to reduce the amount of the cognitive skill worksheets that would be given to me as the homework.

Lisa my dietitian, suggested in the same building the Advanced Medical Group hospital were taking family patients. I inquired about family doctors and I filled the form with the help of Adriene and I submitted my form. I also brought the family doctor form for my son and my husband. After contacting the hospital, first my son and I got registered there, finding a family doctor for each of us. Soon, my husband too found a family doctor in that hospital. Our family got settled in the matter of finding a family doctor.

We also got settled in the new house, after arranging all rooms. I was still engaged in making some or other changes in the home decoration. That was a positive factor, as it was keeping my attention away from the brain injury related problems. I had sometimes occasional visitors at the home that would keep me suggesting some tips about decorating the house.

April 2019

My health was stable, and there was no signal of any imminent issue. However, all the sudden on April 2, when I was working in the garden, I started feeling dizzy. My son was in gym and I decided to wait for him. Meanwhile, I went to bed myself and closed my eyes. After some time, he came from the gym and gave me the medicine that he would always keep in his workbag. After discussing with me, he decided to opt for the medical help. I told him that the next day I had family doctor's appointment at the Advance Medical Group hospital.

It was a psychological advantage as I started feeling relieved to some extend after knowing about the family doctor appointment. My doctor was Dr Robert Natalie, a soft spoken, friendly person and an easily approachable professional. The nurse checked my weight, height etc., as per the primary check procedure. Then, the doctor told me to go for the blood testing. My son had to go through the same procedure, as it was his first visit too. We spent the whole day in the hospital, completing various formalities and essential paperwork.

Later, the therapists informed me that I would get a dietitian as per the Outpatient plan. Perhaps, they wanted me to put more efforts or to have a different approach to improve my health eliminating the diet related problems. I needed to develop the stamina that would allow me to work for the longer period without causing any health issue. I would try to achieve such stamina, but I could not erase the brain injury and its effects altogether.

The hospital called me after four days. The doctor explained my blood report to me, explaining its all aspects and major points. She told me that my blood sugar and bad cholesterol levels had increased. After discussing my eating habits in detail, she pointed out that the health issue might be the result of consuming sweets and red meat in excess. I explained that I included these items in my diet to gain more energy. She removed my misconception about these intakes and alerted that there could be chances of heart stroke, though such possibility was not imminent.

After discussing some other related points, including the supplements that I was taking, she gave me the medications. She also mentioned it to me that she would like to monitor my improvement process by observing the side effects of the given medications. Finally, she assured me of the recovery, and I left the hospital on the positive note.

I went to collect the medicine from the adjoining pharmacy. In the process, I had some cordial talk with the pharmacist Patel, a nice person having the deep professional knowledge. After discussing with me and going through my medication details, he advised me not to consume grapes or grapefruits, as they could nullify the function of the medication. He suggested me to avoid as much as possible the consumption of white bread and sugar in order to get quick and better results.

A week passed in following the received medical instructions. Then as per the scheduled appointment, I visited the family doctor, who delivered the same instructions, though with some modification. After having medical treatment from her, I contacted the dietician. After some discussion, in order to get additional information, she prepared a there-week meal plan for me. She also recommended to do regular exercises suggested by the physio. Confirming the suggestions of the pharmacist Patel, she told me to avoid grapefruits, bananas, pineapples and some other fruits. She told me to have blueberries at least one bowl per day. She advised me to consume some specific vegetables, like red, yellow, and orange pepper, broccoli, spinach, and other leafy greens in profusion. She prohibited me for consuming any sort of fast food. She also mentioned that rice must be completely avoided, and bread must be eaten in the moderation. Some other items, like the hummus were included in my meal plans.

There was a change in my stance too. Earlier, I would refuse to visit the grocery stores mentioning that I would like to visit only fancy stores, like furniture shops and clothes stores. However, now, I started visiting myself to the grocery stores or joining my husband in order to find my desired food items.

Heather, the new therapist had the responsibility of finding a physio for me. She forwarded some options, however she would find it difficult to determine a physio for several reasons. First, given my brain injury issue, she needed to find a physio working in the related field. Second, most physio in that category were already engaged with the patients. Eventually, she found an Indian physio, Rajendeer for me. She told me that he would start regularly visiting shortly.

As the dietician instructed, I visited her to explain the changes I had made in my diet plan. After conducting some check ups on me, she suggested me to increase physio exercises. She assured me that such extended exercises would be safe, given my health conditions. She reminded me that I was fighting against the negative impacts of the brain injury, and as a dietician, she was making all recommendations that were safe for me. She told me to add a short distance walk and some stationary steps in my regular exercise schedule. She cautioned me to change the activities if I found at any point myself stressful while doing any exercise. She also insisted to add the gardening activities in my regular physical movement plan. Overall, she was satisfied with my health improvement.

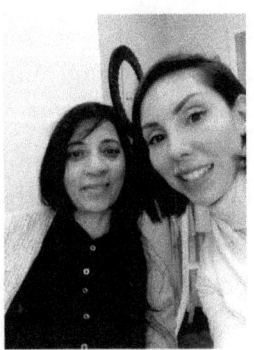

My Dietician

As per the schedule, the new physio, Rajendeer, visited at home. In the formal discussion, he mentioned that his wife was also a physio. He had two lovely young twin daughters, studying in the junior kindergarten. He grudged that some patients would find it difficult to follow his professional directives related to physical exercise, thus they would not achieve the desired improvements. He told me that he would visit once in every two weeks. He demonstrated how to do the neck exercise and told me to perform it everyday as it was very effective in the case of brain injury. I told him that I would feel sleepy after remaining in the sitting position for long. Thus, in addition, he demonstrated some leg exercises to resolve the issue.

The physio also mentioned that the physical activities could also be calculated in the term of the calories burning, a measurable process. On his suggestions, my son bought fit-bit for me. It could calculate the amount of calories burned if we would wear it while doing physical exercise. My son had set the device as per physio's instructions. Thus, I would be able to control the amount of my physical movements accordingly.

May 2019

Finally, it was the beginning of the summer. I always enjoyed the summer as it brought me happy memories. My aspiration from the life was to learn new things, to express my feelings through the creative arts, to explore the world, to visit the new places, and to share the experience of people from different culture. In my childhood, when I saw the picture of the Statue of Liberty in my textbook, I wanted to visit it. Then my father told me that it was in New York, which was far away. In that delicate age, I wanted to travel to New York some time in my life. I would think that by visiting new places, I would gain a collection of information and experience from different sources, which would make me a wiser person leading to a pleasant and content life.

Meanwhile, I had an appointment with the doctor at Parkwood. After completing the routine check up, Dr Sequeira told me that I was doing well. I told him about the medications recommended by the family doctor. He found the entire medication compatible with my health improvement plan. My weight was gradually decreasing under the dietitian supervision. She had told me to keep checking my body weight regularly. Thus, I bought a weight machine, and put it in my bedroom. My husband would never believe in measuring the body weight. For him a strong body and sustaining stamina were enough. However, watching constant and steady progress in losing unwanted weight would make me more positive in putting efforts towards the health improving goal.

I went to the family doctor and per the schedule that I got the last month. She checked my reports, and other details. Then she said that I would be sent for diabetic seminar if my condition would not improve, though she also added that it was not needed to be done immediately. I thought that I was on the way of being a diabetic patient, an additional problem. However, she declined of having such possibility at least at that stage. My dietitian gave me a chart about the diet control plan.

The therapists would mention that I needed to divert my attention towards the house decoration and gardening to have some change from the routine life and to have additional physical movements in different manner. They also told me to be extrovert and express my feelings, thoughts, and aspirations by connecting with other creative activities, like art making. I was already doing some artwork. I wanted to do gardening, but the first half of the month was not favourable.

In the second half of the month, the semi-summer like weather allowed me for implementing gardening activities. I would go to the nearby store with the therapists and would keep buying several gardening related items in order to getting prepared for my gardening venture. In that attempt, I learned more about gardening.

The therapists kept visiting but that was more a welcoming schedule than a dull classroom exercise. Since I would do more gardening and artwork, I would feel content from inside leaving the brain injury impact at some corner of my mind. The weather was turning more pleasant with passing of each day, so that was a bonus point. However, I would feel sometime paranoid with the unexplained feeling of probable health issue. It was like the feeling of some unknown shadow following me to prevent me from moving forward. I could try to leave the brain injury behind, but the same would not allow me to live alone.

June 2019

The month started with the commencement of the pleasant weather. The air was warmer, grass was greener, and sky was clearer. It was almost like the Indian summer, though with two noteworthy differences. First, the trees were full of leaves here whereas in India the trees would start shedding their leaves in the summer. Second, in India, the temperature would frequently be above 40 degrees Celsius, which could not be called pleasant.

As a teacher, I could feel the difference of the scenario too. At the end of the month, here the schools were going to be closed whereas in India, in the first week of the month, the school would start. Besides, 7 June would be the official opening date for Monsoon, the rainy season, in India. Thus, I would have a psychological picture for this month – several kids going to school wearing coloured raincoats.

I recalled that, in childhood, we would not sleep in the afternoon, though our parents would like us sleeping so that we could not wander in the hot sun, which could easily make us suffer from the sunstroke. After getting reprimanded from my mother, we would close our eyes for a while and once the mother turned her back, we would start playing. We children would put our heads into a bucket full of water. My mother would rush towards us and would stop us from doing so. She would tell us how dangerous it could be for us. At that point in time, I did not understand her. However, now after I have become a mother, I can understand her perspective.

My son's birthday was on 13 June. I prepared his favourite dishes for him. However, he had busy schedule now. Earlier, he would go to the school, but now he would go to the office to work and was also preparing for the upcoming exams too. Nevertheless, my motherly approach did not change. I would still wait and be happy to see him when he would come back from the office. I would feel the same happiness when he would come back from the school after the long day. In India, he would have his school vacations in June.

However, on his every birthday, I would give him a handmade art piece. On such occasions, he would gratefully recall that I took the required care of his studies even in his early classes, so that his education foundation got cemented. I remembered that I would give him repeated practice of writing and reading that improved his study habits and knowledge too. Since I was strict, my husband was lenient with him considering him in his delicate age to be treated with affectionate and soft hands. However, the treatment, I gave my son for his studies, was now being received by me. I was going through the same repeated procedure of completing homework, solving the worksheets, and performing the physio exercises, guided by the therapists. Indeed, the entire procedure was prolonged and hence was irritating. However, the procedure was much needed to bring the expected physical strength and cognitive improvement in me. Therefore, I needed to continue that useful process. To keep my interest in that process and my daily life intact, I would also watch television serials. They may not have the facts like science or history textbooks, but they would teach about human behavior a lot. The more serials you watch, the more you know about real people around. You need to remain updated in order to fight against the negative psychological impact of the brain injury.

I had the dietitian appointment after a couple of days. I went to the clinic with the unsure mind because every time I would get some or other treatment instructions after finding some deficiency. However, during this visit, I received only complementary feedback. She told me that I was getting improved. Commending my constant efforts, she advised me to follow the increased exercise plan. To my relief, she mentioned that there would be no additional protein.

At Parkwood, on 17 June, I had an appointment with Dr Sequeira. It was a short meeting. He found all reports fine. He allowed me to increase my outdoor activities as I was not getting tired within the short span of physical movements. He also recommended to increase the process of communication with people around. Thus, by the end of the month, because of all positive happenings around me, and also my encouraging communication with the doctors, therapists and dietitians, I realized that I was moving towards the point of recovery, if not complete then partially, from the setback of the brain injury. I also realized that the brain injury might keep bringing different moods - anxiety, despair, loss, shock, and so on. I needed to be in self-control to overcome these momentary issues. The professionals could only assist me. Nonetheless, I had to fight the real battle.

July 2019

The month began with the Canada Day, 1 July. I had been always curious and enthusiastic about the national celebrations. In India, in my childhood, I would enjoy wearing new clothes on 15 August, the Independence Day, and 26 January, the Republic Day. My elder siblings would go to the school, and me in my new frock, holding their hands, would walk with my tint feet on the familiar roads of the colony to go to the school. Although, I was not old enough to go to school yet. Later, when I got admitted in the school, I would joyfully rush for participating in various cultural activities. There were several events in the school and would almost watch them all. During my later student life in the school and then college, I would like to watch movies in theatres with my friends. I had seen several Amitabh Bachchan movies on the first day first show on such national celebration occasions. It was a childlike enthusiasm, but that was me.

When I started working in the school, the matter of the national day celebration became official. I would take interest not only because it was my duty but also because I had personal interest. True that I would have to bear more responsibilities, but it was never purely duty for me. I would also enjoy working on the preparation of the event and would ensure that other teachers to work for the same objective. I was fortunate for having teachers' support in that matter, so I would find myself enjoying the students' activities.

In Canada, before suffering from the brain injury, I would like to go to different places to watch the celebrations on Victoria Day and

Canada Day. In 2007, just after my arrival in Canada, I went to the Grand Bend to watch the fireworks. That day I felt it was very cold, although 1 July was a cold day for having thick clouds overhead. While going to Grand Bend, we kept watching with astonishment the green farmlands, windmills, passing hills, colourful gardens, grazing cattle, like cows and sheep, running horses in the yards, and county road settings. It was all new for me. Finally, when we arrived at the Grand Bend, first we stopped at a nearby beach. It was turning golden in the setting sunlight. There were several boats tied around. The cottages were beautiful. However, it was too cold to go into the water. We marvelled at the visitors' courage. In that cold weather, they were wandering around in shorts. Ironically, the fire works got cancelled because conditions were not optimal. It was a disappointment, but we enjoyed our first outing in Canada.

However, now, I had to watch Canada Day fireworks from my home. We could watch it from our Oxford window, so I did not need to go outdoors. Because of my brain injury, I could not bear the noisy and crowded places. Unlike my past choices, now I started preferring the peaceful environment. Nevertheless, it was not alarming as my desire of watching such events was still alive.

Now, the weather was warmer and sunny. I was glad that it was suitable for gardening. I had already brought enough gardening material from the nearby store while visiting with my therapists. One of my neighbours told me that the previous tenants did not take proper care of our garden thus we need to take care of the weed control. With hard work and investment of lot of time, I cleared and then decorated the garden. Then I sent its pictures to my son who was then working in his office. In the lunch time his coworkers saw the pictures and said that it was the job of a professional. That compliment made me very happy.

On 4 July, my son took me to SunFest at Victoria Park. I saw the current prime minister, Mr. Justin Trudeau there. He was appearing fit and handsome. I was far away, so I could not hear his speech properly. Nevertheless, I was happy for seeing the prime minister of our country.

I had a dream since childhood to see a current prime minister. In India, I never got the opportunity. However, now my wish was fulfilled.

On 13 July, Sunday, it was my birthday. My son had bought pearl earrings for me. My husband told me to buy anything of my choice. I bought a model of a ship, a decorative piece from the nearby antique shop. My husband came back from the work and we all went for a bank appointment. It was a time-consuming meeting. I felt that I could not focus around because of the lack of concentration, energy and stamina. Thus, we straight came back home after the meeting and celebrated my birthday at home.

During this month, it would be mostly sunny and clear weather, so I would keep walking in the neighbourhood. I could meet everyday many other walkers from the nearby areas. We would wish to each other. It would be a brief communication but still it was effective in increasing my confidence. In addition, some kids were so familiar that they would keep waving at me. I would feel that I was still connected with the society despite of not being in the workforce. I got my blood report by the end of the month, which was normal. The doctor told me to keep taking the medications as recommended. I had to continue the medications for the next there months. I consoled myself that I had won the first front, and if I kept improving in the same way, I would get rid of the medication forever.

The next appointment was with the dietitian. After going through all my reports, she told me that I needed to consume fish. Initially, I told her that I did not like fish in my diet. Upon hearing that she told me to choose between fish and the supplements. I did not want more medications. Therefore, I preferred fish over the supplements. She told me to have salmon fish three times in a week. I was happy that I successfully avoided one more regular medical intake.

The rest of the month was eventless. I had all therapists' regular classes, but no more medical appointments. I started feeling from inside that I was on the path of improvement, though occasional hiccups in the form of mental fatigue and physical weakness were there. However, undoubtably, I was far better than I was two months before.

August 2019

It was the last month of the summer, and then it would be Fall. I thought vulnerably that seasons kept changing even if you do not like such changes. Summer would be always special for me, as my family would always like to go for outing in this season. However, in the last couple of summers, we could not go for many short or long outings because of my brain injury and its treatment plans.

My therapy classes were going well, without any complication, I mean no further medical check ups or additional training schedule. The therapists gave me off for a week; there would be classes in all first three weeks and then the last week was off. I decided to utilize this opportunity. We went to Pinery suddenly without having any elaborated planning. We straight went for paddle boating, but I noticed that it was not that scary this time as it was the last time. I enjoyed the view around. Being a Botany and Zoology student, the vegetation and creatures under the water were special attraction for me. We spent two hours boating, and most of time my husband kept paddling as usual. After all, he was the most eager one to visit here. Then we collected a lot of stones and pebbles from the beach to decorate my drawing room and the garden. My husband had already brought six bags of pebbles from a farming field on the last weekend. I joked that passerby must be enjoying the view after watching him collecting the pebbles for two hours. Anyway, after collecting two bags of pebbles. We went in the recreation area and the father and son bought ice cream cones. They did not make any comment at all, but the way they were making faces while eating was indicating that the treat was not much delicious. Had I ordered it, I would have to hear a lot; fortunately, I did not do that mistake. When it started turning dark, we came back to our home.

I had an appointment for eye check up on 10 August. It was just a regular check up and was not recommended by a therapist. The doctor assured me that there was no damage in eyes despite of my increasing blood sugar. I was content to hear that. All the therapists were following the schedule. However, one more therapist got added in the team. She was a social worker, Julia. Perhaps, she was there to co-ordinate all therapy classes and their findings. Later, in that week, Lani informed me that she had found a full-time position in July itself. Thus, during this month, she needed to join the job duties. She further explained that Jenifer, the new therapist would replace her. On her schedule, Jenifer, visited. She was a rehabilitation therapist and a nice lady. She told me that she would also conduct the classes of cognitive skills. She outlined the probable plans for me and also explained how to prepare for it. Heather, the therapist, conveyed that she was going on the maternity leave after this month. She gave me some practice worksheets in advance to keep the continuity. She also brought her replacement, Kevin. Although I was not keen for attempting the driving test immediately, the therapists told me to have a look at the plan. Accordingly, I checked the vehicle arranged for my driving test. After boarding into the driver's seat for a while, I told them that vehicle was not comfortable for me. Also, I did not have the required stamina for the test. I informed the therapists that I would take the driving test in the next April. Perhaps, they had assessed it beforehand, so they agreed with my decision and forwarded their recommendations to the decision-making team.

Later in that week, the speech therapist explained to me that to be a part of the workforce, or even to carry out my everyday responsibilities, I needed to be confident in the communication skills. She agreed that partially my problem was my limited hearing capacity. However, I knew as she did too that my root problem was the cognitive skill loss because of the brain injury. Under her guidance, I was practicing for checking my phone communication skill. In addition, she would take me in the Farm Boy to check if I could handle communication in the noisy places.

I would still get anxious after staying in the noisy places for a while. Noticing my disturbed mindset, all therapists advised me to be seated in the garden for getting relieved. They had also mentioned that the growing plants, blooming flowers and spreading greenery around would have healing effect on me. Meanwhile, I started watching Nach Baliye season 9, a Hindi dance show, produced by the Hindi movie star, Salman Khan. In the current episode, one of the themes was Women Empowerment. I found the show quite inspiring. I thought that I could not go back to work for the long time because of my brain injury, but I could still achieve my previous skills by putting forward my best efforts. In that show, a participant had mentioned that the process of self expression, like conveying the inner struggle and feelings to others, was a constructive step from getting away from the health setback.

However, this "speaking of personal experience" was a calculated risk-taking process. I could expose my inner personality, but I could also help others in having a different perspective on the suffering and the recovery. I had several contradictory thoughts, but finally I decided that for keeping myself into a constructive work, I would use my diary for narrating my story of recovery from the brain injury.

I discussed my idea with Adrienne. She inspired me to focus on it. She added that it would give me mental exercise and would be good for my cognitive skills. My objective would be to inspire other patients for putting more efforts towards the recovery process while enjoying the present life. However, I needed to clear some cobwebs and talk to some persons close to me before starting the venture.

My friend Shubhangi's birthday was on 16 July. I contacted her to convey my good wishes. In the discussion, I told her my intention of writing my experience. She was excited about it. She reminded me that during my student life, I would write essays and got some prizes too. She told me to restart my writing practice. Then I talked to Sameena, who also inspired me to write down my experience, stating that it would be inspirational for other patients. Once I determined to pen my experience, I also decided that I would hide the real identities of the characters appearing in my narration by using pseudonyms. However, in some cases, I needed to use the real characters too. Thus, I had initiated the process of getting their consents for mentioning their identities. I was glad that only in the short period, I got approval from all characters to quote their names in my story.

On 30 August, for congratulating my previous colleagues from the school in India, I had contacted my Indian friends. Among them, Bhagyashree sent me a video of a physically challenged sportswoman. In an accident, she got her one leg amputated. However, she went back to the competitive games after having a wooden leg. The same case was of Sudhachandran, an Indian dancer and actress. She had lost her leg in an accident, but with the wooden leg, she made a comeback and was still working in movies. I recalled that in 1996, during my pregnancy period, I wrote the Master of Arts exam for three hours. I asked myself why I could not have the same stamina now. I assured myself that I was not suffering from any memory loss, and it was only a case of cognitive loss, so my determination could bring me back into the action. Another lady, Julie Sawchuk from Ontario, appeared as an inspiration figure for me. She was riding her bike, when a car hit her. She was airlifted to Victoria Hospital. She went through multiple surgeries and remained hospitalized for several months. She was paralyzed and is now wheelchair ridden. However, she faced all adversities with determination and emerged as an inspiration for other struggling patients by engaging in several constructive work and activities. I also had the example of Terry Fox, a Canadian athlete. His one leg was amputated due to cancer tissue. Instead of getting disappointed, he became a cancer research activist.

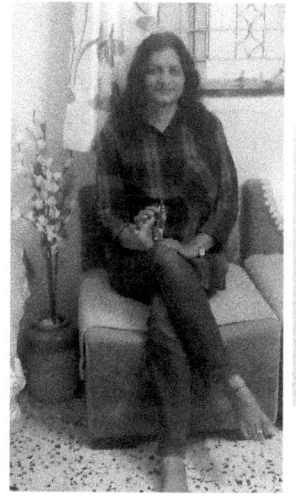

My Friend Shubangi

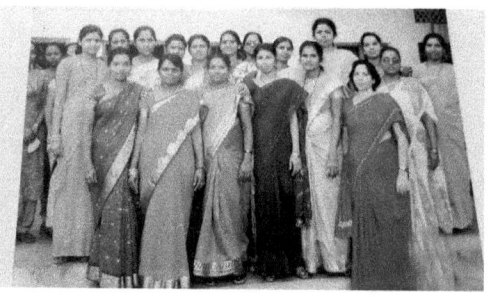

My Staff from India

Meanwhile, Julia, the therapist, who was pregnant, informed that she would quit the job. She told me that she had a horse farmhouse. She further explained that some patients like to receive the therapy treatment by doing horse riding. Thus, she would run her therapy classes from her home. With my good wishes, I gave a gift for her would be baby, as I gave to Susan and Heather on their pregnancy leave.

I contemplated that Julia was focussed in the changing conditions too. She was focussing on her life mission and was staying steadfast to it. By sharing my experience, I could contribute in removing at least a small part of that unfairness to make life somewhat fair for some people around me.

September 2019

On 5 September, when I called some of my friends in India, I was reminded that the celebration of Teachers' Day was going on. I recollected that I would also participate in several teachers' activities while I was working in the school. I was good in co-curricular activities, though I was not an average singer. But with other teachers, in the group singing, I would also sing qawwali and act with other teachers. Most of our teachers would have to carry multiple responsibilities of profession at the school and of families at their homes. Thus, such merrymaking time was a boon for us to relieve the expected stress.

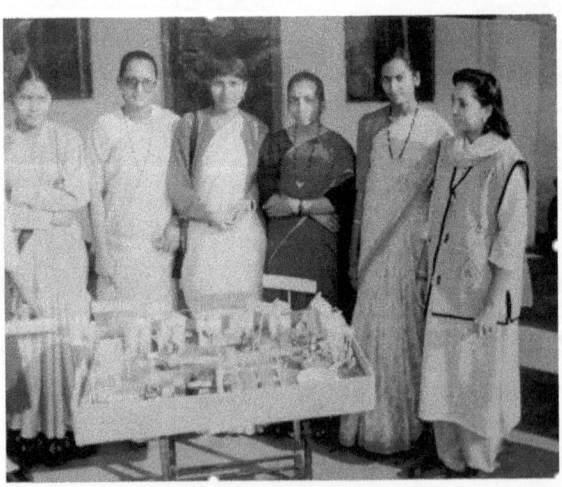

Science Exhibition

My conversation with my Indian friends reminded me that I visited my hometown the ten years before in the same month. My siblings in India were surprised how I was travelling on my own. Since I was the youngest one, they all were quite protective about me. They had another reason for getting surprised. In fact, I had never left my family for a single day or night, but this time I was away for fifty-two days on my own. It was a mixed strange feeling, as on one side, I was enthusiastic for visiting my hometown and my loving siblings, relatives, and my close friends, after a long time but on the other side, I was disappointed also for not being with my family for so extended period. Initially, I would feel pleased when my school going nephews and nieces would proudly tell their classmates that their "Canadian Aunt" was at home, or when the teacher friends would curiously ask about my life in Canada.

As Julia, the social worker, informed me before, it was her last class in the middle of the month. Before leaving, she gave me some tips to follow whenever I had negative feelings. I knew that I was going to miss her. She was replaced by another social worker, Jennifer, who was a nice lady too. The appointment with the dietitian was a delight, as she said that all reports were normal, and more significantly, she declared that my body weight was in the optimal range.

The weather started turning cooler, so I needed to stop gardening, my favourite activity. That was a setback for my outdoor activities, though I had arranged several indoor plants. I was glad to see them growing. Anyway, after losing the option of gardening, I was looking for some identical option, when Kevin, the therapist, informed me that the Northwest Resource Centre agreed to accommodate me for volunteering. He also told me that I would get morning hours to work there. I had previously informed the Centre that I could not work in the afternoon timings that the Centre had offered earlier. This was because I would get tired later in the day. I was approved by doctors at Parkwood for volunteering at Northwest Resource center.

There was an outdoor volunteering event in the city, Reforest London on 21 September. My son volunteered with me in planting trees near the London airport. It was a lot of fun for me and my son. Even though the task got tiring towards the end, we enjoyed planting trees a lot. I felt very good as it was similar to my previous gardening activities. In the break, the organizing committee provided us with ice cream cones. After the event was complete, both me and my son were very tired. It was a day well spent. I recalled that I did the similar activities in India as a teacher. We all science teachers were participating, wearing green saris. The students also got involved. However, there was a big difference. I would work independently in those days, but now for planting, I needed to take my son's help. Perhaps, that physical inability turned me a little emotional. So, I told him to show my planted trees to my grandchildren. Also, I explained him the importance of plants. I told him that he would get oxygen by the indoor plants that I had nursed at home.

The next day, I told the therapists about my volunteering at Reforest London. However, I also confessed that I got tired soon. One therapist suggested me to carry dry fruits the next time while performing outdoor activities so that I could get the required energy supply constantly. After planting the trees, I felt that my utility was still relevant. I was still able to do physically strenuous work. In a way, volunteering at Reforest London rejuvenated me and convinced me that I still had the required skills in me.

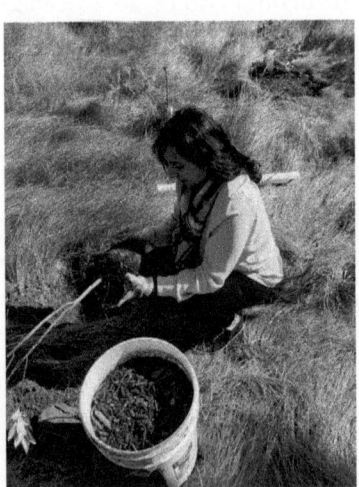

Reforest London: Volunteering for first time after injury

October 2019

On the 3rdof October, I went for a blood test. Anyway, after a couple of days, I went to my family doctor, who told me that the blood report was normal, thus no further medication was needed. I felt relieved with this information. Meanwhile, Kevin, the occupational therapist took me for volunteering interview on 7th October. After a brief interview, which was mainly meant for a formal introduction, the volunteer coordinator told me that another volunteer, Jennatte, would guide me in preparing to resume volunteer's duties. She also told me that I had been allotted the morning session to work.

On the same day, I had an appointment with the dietitian in the noon. She found my body weight and medical conditions balanced. She also told me that although I did not need any further appointment for having good health condition, I have to visit one more time to complete the formalities. She suggested me to increase physio exercises if I found my weight going up. During that week, my husband suggested that we buy two tall chairs for the bedroom window from where we could have the panoramic view of oxford and entire city. I was surprised because he would normally avoid buying new things unless it was absolutely required. He would say when people buy, they think of their social status instead of their requirement and after buying an item they find it useless within ten days. Anyway, we went for buying the chairs on 12 October.

After looking into three shops, we narrowed on one chair, which was simple, tall, and suitable for our purpose. However, he suggested that we should look into a big shop, having a wide collection of chairs. It was located at the Exeter road. I agreed after knowing that it was not far away. While driving towards the shop, we passed in front of the Montcalm school. That made me recall my accident. I went to the school on the day of the accident and talked to the vice principal. She explained some basics to me and then told me to inform her if students would create any problem. Everything was going on well, till reached to the stairs and then it was all dark for me. My train of thoughts was broken when we arrived at the big store. I had never seen such wide collection of chairs. All sort of sizes, shapes, and structures were available there. My head started reeling after looking at so many chairs. Finally, we decided to order the chair that we previously selected.

After a couple of days, I went to the Parkwood hospital with Jennifer who was my rehabilitation therapist. The hospital building and the staff were reassuring. However, when I saw the patients, I started feeling nervous. I started feeling that I might not get improved. However, I could also understand those patients' feelings. Thus, I wish that they should get recovered soon.

In my therapy classes, Kevin would give me cognitive skill practice in Sherwood Mall. He was very nice and soft spoken. He was very

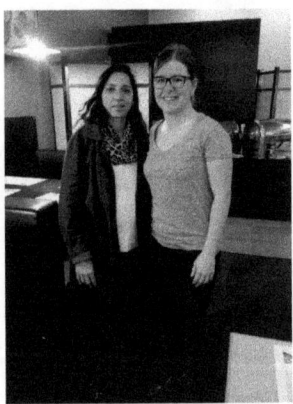

My Rehabilitation therapist,
Jennifer H

friendly and trying his best to help me in handling the stress of noisy places. It was an essential part of getting me prepared for joining the professional work.

Soon, I started volunteering at the Northwest Resource Centre. It was the part of my therapies to come out from the home and involve in the community. I was getting so many instructions and so much feedback that I felt like I was starting from zero. Such feelings naturally surface when your working conditions get suddenly changed. In India, I was well set in my job, and rarely would receive instructions for changing my work pattern. In Canada too, I was comfortably working from a long time. However, now I needed to learn everything from the beginning. It was not much comfortable feeling.

Another volunteer, Jennate was also working there. She was very nice. She would keep suggesting me how to perform various tasks. I assessed that the work was not difficult but to continue with the required stamina was difficult. Mostly I would find myself out of energy after an hour's work. On the first day, the volunteer coordinator asked me which task I would like to do. I would prefer to work on the computer. I told them that I did not operate a computer from long time thus, I might be slow in completing the computer tasks.

It was the election period. On 20 October, I went to vote with my family. We voted almost ten days before the scheduled voting date, because my family was busy after that. It was a feeling of fulfilment to exercise the voting right. After voting, we went to a nearby small farmer market to take pictures with the big pumpkin, which were meant for Halloween. I wanted to take the picture with pumpkin during the last year itself, but I missed because of my relatively fresh brain injury.

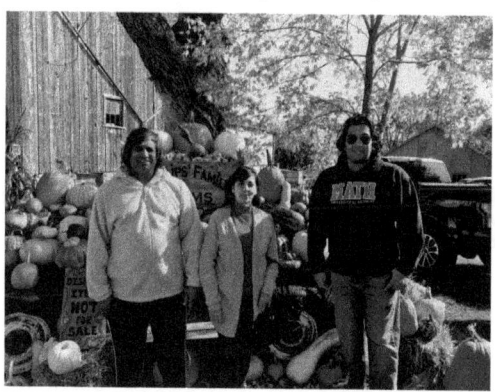

Visiting Pumpkin Farm for Halloween

Adrienne was frequently asking me about my volunteering experience. I told her that the work was not difficult, but I felt tired within an hour. She told me that such tiredness might occur because I did not have the habit of sitting for long time at one spot. She told me that eventually, I would not feel tired. On 31 October, on Halloween Day, lot of kids from our neighbourhood, visited our home and got candies.

I was happy that I did not miss to participate in the festival. There is nothing more pleasing in the world than to watch happy kids. Their happy faces and innocent smiles bring heaven on the earth.

November 2019

I was volunteering every week with the help of the therapists, and started feeling comfortable with the work, the place and the people around me. Kevin suggested me to increase my volunteering hours with the passing of the days. Meanwhile the speech therapist, Coney, had a short meeting with me. She praised me for my positive approach. To keep myself positive and engaged, I started working on my idea of sharing my experience with others, especially with the patients, in order to motivate them to remain positive about recovering. The therapists assured me that they would help me with editing and publishing my story. However, sometimes, I was finding it difficult to focus on the writing task.

Once I could focus constantly in difficult situations. I was in the San Diego zoo with my son and we were riding in Skyfari, an aerial tram. My son was scared to go on the aerial tram as he was afraid of heights, however, I was focused on helping him overcome his fear. To keep his focus away from the height, I started humming different sounds; by the time the ride was finished, he was laughing whole heartedly. That made me feel very good. Whenever I remember that incident, it brings a smile to my face.

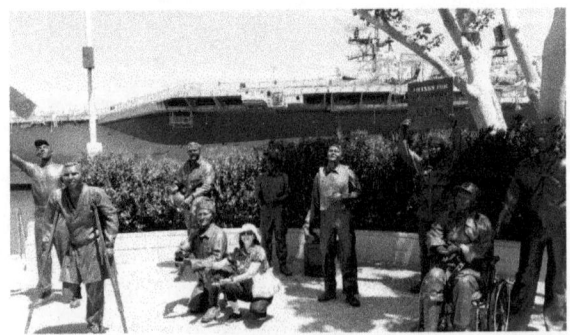

At San Diego

To improve my focus, I started playing table tennis regularly with my family. It was interesting to learn new techniques of the game and put all efforts to win. My son was a good player and my husband was not bad either, but I started showing some fighting spirit. Eventually, I started to defeat both my son and husband consistently.

During the citizenship oath in Canada, the minister said that we had to keep a balance between the customs of our home country and the traditions of Canada. He suggested that we should not forget our roots, but it was also important to follow the laws of the land. I agreed with him. Thus, I value both highly: the Republic Day of India, where I wear a new sari, and the Remembrance Day, where I tag myself with a poppy. I like to take interest in and remain curious about what is going on around me.

To remain active, I was suggested by my therapist to join a gym. She said that the physiotherapist will be with me in order to help me practice, however, after doing some exercises, I found that I could not bend down on the treadmill. I tried hard but I would feel my head spinning whenever I did so. I also realized that I could only workout in the mornings as I would lose my stamina and feel tired in the later part of the day.

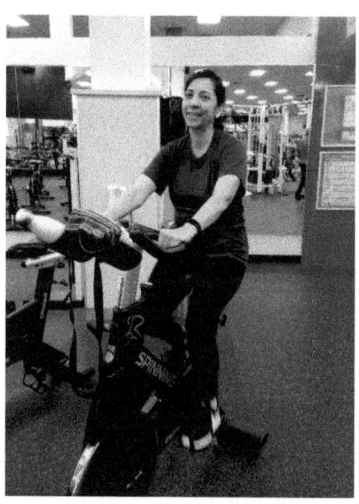

Riding exercise bike

I told the physiotherapist and the social worker about the frequent nervousness that I felt. They told me to do breathing exercises to improve my concentration when I would feel nervous. Similarly, on their advice, I started doing basic math in mind to strengthen my cognitive skills. I started feeling somewhat better, however the frequent nervousness would still be there because of the uncertainty of my future. Then, one day I was with the therapist in a store, buying some items for my living room. On the back of the receipt, there was a code number, that needed to be entered into the system with some feedback, slogan, or caption lines. There would be a draw and I could win a lucky prize. My family mostly ignored that proposition, for two reasons. Firstly, the process was time consuming, and secondly, there would be thousands of entries, so winning chances were extremely slim. However, I submitted my entry and won the prize. I was very happy with this unexpected outcome. I concluded that success never routinely comes to us. We have to take steps forward towards success in order to achieve it. If we want something, then we need to stretch our hand in that direction. Our chances may be slim, but if we do not even try to reach towards our goal, we will never be able to get it. We miss 100% of the shots we never take.

I reassured myself that in this new life with different activities, I need to remain hopeful for a better future. In this tough time, I need to love my limited capacities. I need to keep faith in my efforts for achieving a better life. I must value what I have. I must accept that my life has changed, and this situation is still better than facing a tragic end: an end that I would never want for anyone. I am happy with whatever I have and will be pleased in putting more efforts for achieving whatever life may bring me next. For me, the greatest accomplishment is in rising again after you fall.

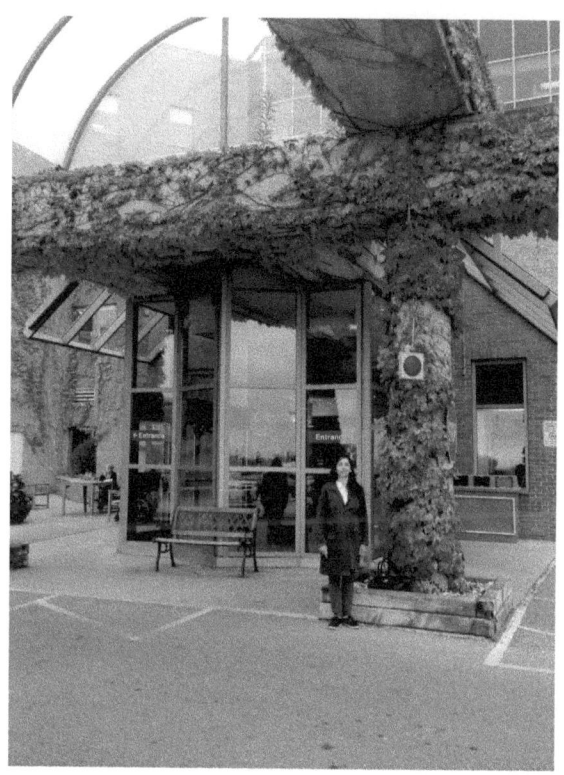

At Parkwood after rising

ACKNOWLEDGMENTS

Enhancing the most one can be is merely not possible without professional help and the active support of others. My journey through Victoria hospital to rehabilitation at Parkwood was accomplished with expert doctors, loving family, friends and professional who dragged me along, boosted me up and washed off when I fell, and sometimes took me on their shoulders.

My debts of gratefulness are enormous and due to many.

Foremost to my son, Sharon whose positive energy, patience, and talent in organising me and editing my work made my writing of this book is possible. His contribution to my well being can not be described or measured. whose untiring energy, and patience boosted me up.

My husband, Vikar whose positive energy, patience, and talent in organising and editing my work made my writing of this book is possible.

I wouldn't be here with the gracious help of the following individuals:

Dr. Kelly Voget
Dr. Keith Sequeira
Dr. Mumtaz Alam
Dr. Mackenzie
The amazing staff of Victoria hospital
The amazing staff of Parkwood Institute team

Dr. Natalie Roberts
Stephanie Muir
Connie Ferri
Jillian Kuepfer
Melissa Fielding
Allison Lawlor
Sarah McLean
Lorra Hanley
Karley Charrette
Chris Fraser
Beb Gibbons
April Zehr
Sarah Carroll
Lisa Spriet
Thames Valley District School Board Officials
Grace Rogers
Staff at Montcalm school
Officials from Work Social Insurance Board
Afroz Khan
Razia Hakim
Javed Sabir
Shabana Pathan
Subhangi Urkude
Maha Noor Alam
Sameena Alvi
Oiwai Chau (April Chau)
Ebrahim Zaveri
Anju Dube
Lalita Walke
Asma Khan
Sunita Kamble
Vanita Inmulwar
Vandana Mojariya
Naheed Imtiaz

Fatimah Sikandar
Joo Young Lee
Adrienne Bulhoes
Lani Saarkoppel
Heather
Kevin Tyrer
Suzi
Susan
Rajendeer
Jennifer Hambleton
Julia Resendes
Jennifer Arthur
Hemang Sheth
Staff at Checker taxi department
Jeanette Kilduff
Amani Radha
Christina Bocora
Officials at North West Resource London
Indie Publishing Group

Lightning Source UK Ltd.
Milton Keynes UK
UKHW010634070121
376597UK00002B/42